Don't eat your Veggies

Same foods can be beneficial or harmful depending on one's Chejil

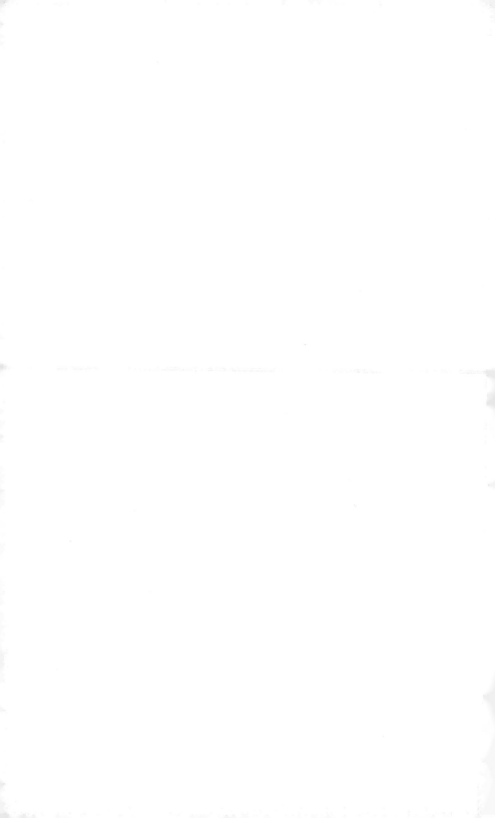

DON'T EAT YOUR VEGGIES

Same foods can be beneficial or harmful depending on one's Chejil

by **Byung Chan Song Lac.**

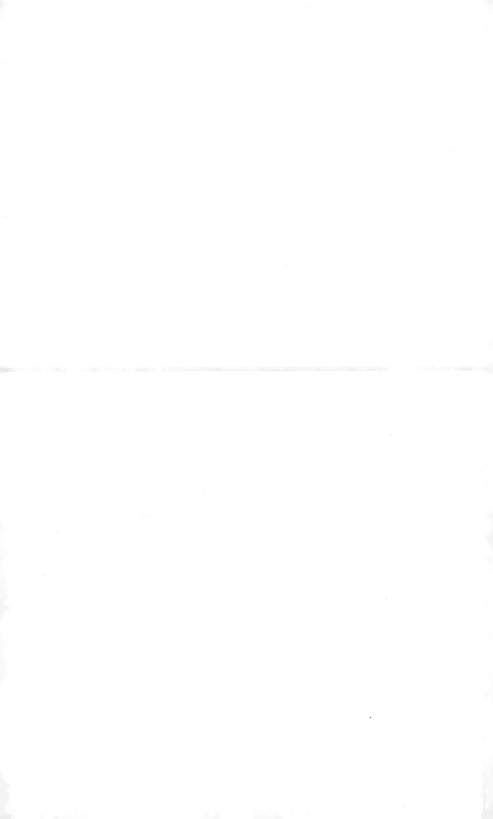

Preface

When I encountered *Chejil* (Constitution) Medicine and applied it in my practice, I discovered that treatment was amazingly fast and accurate. As a result, I am forever indebted to and greatly appreciative of Yi Jae Ma, founder of *Sahsahng* Medicine, and Kwon Do Won, founder of Eight *Chejil* (Constitution) Medicine. I cannot begin to express the wonder when *Chejil* practice effectively treated symptoms that standard medical practices could not. Moreover, I witnessed countless occasions when the principles of *Chejil* refuted erroneous theories of modern medical practice. So, I eagerly desired to inform the general public of the medical misconceptions that they had in order to encourage better decisions for healthier lives. However, I feel that the right time has come for me to share with you some of my writings, which, until now, I did not feel I was fully prepared to do.

"Results judge the value of theories." I particularly enjoy this phrase and use it frequently. My sincere hope is that this book will help you maintain a healthy body, and I believe truly that this book will be tremendously helpful.

B. C. Song LAC

Contents

....

III. Chejil and Nutrition Products

IV. Chejil and Diets

V. CHEJIL AND SICKNESS

VI. CHEJIL AND LIFESTYLE

VII. TAE YANG IN YI JAE MA

Health and Long Life With Chejil Medicine: How to Stay Healthy

People are always concerned about, and expend a great amount of time worrying about, their health and how to live a long and healthy life. Upon entering a bookstore, there are entire sections on health issues and even bestsellers on topics such as overcoming cancer, disease prevention and treatment, and dieting. The topics are endless. Many people buy and follow the book's guidelines, but the truth of the matter is that many are not satisfied with the results.

For every person whose health improved through diet or vitamins, there may be another for whom those things did not work. That person may have suffered various side effects from dieting or taking vitamins. Some people benefit from folk remedies while others do not, or may even experience side effects. For others, certain food items or nutrients may trigger upset stomach, acid reflux, diarrhea, headaches, and/or skin reactions. Hard liquor may be fine for some, but beer might cause diarrhea. Some people drink coffee at all times of the day and are not affected by it, while others would be up all night with even a sip. There are those who feel refreshed and energized after sitting in a hot sauna while others might feel more tired and sleepy afterwards.

Nowadays, numerous supplemental dietary products abound. Ads claims practically promise eternal youth.

Some ads show "before" and "after" images claiming a near-miraculous change. Though it may be true that some people do experience change from dietary products, there are countless others who have experienced little to no change following the use of those same supplements or folk remedies. Instead, negative side effects may have followed.

Some time ago, research reported that drinking 3 to 4 cups of coffee a day was good for the heart. However, recent research has reported that coffee is stressful to the heart. Recently, breathing exercises have become popular, but even with this, some have benefited while others have not. Antibiotics, penicillin, aspirin, and even gold crowns are effective for some yet cause side effects or even allergic reactions in others. Why is it that what is good for some only causes side effects or allergic reactions in others?

Take, for instance, the flagship supplemental dietary product: the vitamin. Vitamins were first developed and mass produced in the 1960s. Makers claimed that because vitamins were organic compounds, they would have no side effects, regardless of dosage. They claimed that vitamins could only be good for the body. There were even claims that in the near future, a day would come when people could cease to eat any meals and instead take some vitamin pills. In those days, vitamins were talked about everywhere from the media to schools to companies. Looking at it now, over forty years later, what are feelings towards vitamins? Research currently reveals side effects and negative aspects of vitamin consumption. As a result, since several years ago, researchers have tried to develop natural herbal supplements to reduce side effects, but to no avail. Recently, the U.S. Department of Health and Human Services reported that vitamins were neither helpful nor harmful.

Several years ago, an unbelievable vitamin C-mania blew through South Korea. One professor from Seoul National University appeared on a national television program and proclaimed, "Vitamin C effectively increases the body's natural immune system to ward off many diseases such as high blood pressure, heart disease, and stroke." After this program aired, nearly every person in South Korea went on a vitamin C diet. This fad, however, lasted only a brief moment as a research team from the University of Pennsylvania reported that although vitamin C positively functions to block genes from being damaged, it also produces toxic elements that damage genes using fat oxides in the body.

Therefore, the question remains: How can consumers receive the positive effects of vitamin C without negative side effects? The answer lies in what Yi Jae Ma, the founder of *Sahsahng* Medicine, and Kwon Do Won, the founder of Eight *Chejil* Medicine, believed—each person is born with a certain *Chejil*, which is a particular innate organization of strong and weak internal organs. In one word, everybody's *Chejil* is different. These differences may explain the inconsistent effects of such things as vitamins and remedies, and why some things work better for some than others. To answer the question of how one's health can be improved, one must discover his or her *Chejil* and maintain a diet that is specific to that *Chejil*. The same principles would extend to supplemental dietary products. What, then, is good for one's health? It all depends on one's *Chejil*.

I

CHEJIL

"Know your Chejil, know your health."

What is *Chejil*?

Chejil is part of everyday conversation for many Koreans. People often talk about it in terms of opposites: weak *Chejil*, healthy *Chejil*, fat *Chejil*, skinny *Chejil*, alkaline *Chejil* and acidic *Chejil*, or even about certain occupational *Chejil*, dispositional or indispositional *Chejil*, allergic *Chejil*, and so on.

In *Chejil* medicine, *Chejil* refers to the distribution of people into several patterns according to the particular organization of strong and weak internal organs within each person, which include the liver, gall bladder, heart, small intestines, spleen, stomach, lungs, large intestines, kidney, and bladder. The combination of strong and weak organs makes up the different patterns. Because the strength and weakness of the internal organs are different, each person's physiology, pathology of disease, physical appearance, and personality are different according to one's *Chejil*. In other words, depending on whether a certain internal organ's function is strong or weak, its influence will depend upon the specific function of the organ. Its influence can range from physical to emotional to physiological. This is the reason why diets, supplemental dietary products, and vitamins produce different effects on different people. It is also the reason why medications or acupuncture treatments must be specialized according to each individual. Moreover, the body takes on different physical characteristics according to its *Chejil* as the body grows and matures according to the strengths and weaknesses of the various internal organs. One of the principles of *Chejil* medication is that one's *Chejil* remains constant from birth until death. For example, if one's kidneys are the weakest among the other internal organs, then the kidneys will remain the weakest organ for the rest of one's life.

The idea of *Chejil* has been around throughout history. In the west, Hippocrates proposed the theory of four humors (blood, phlegm, yellow bile, and black bile) in the body. Galen built upon the theory of four humors and proposed his own four temperaments (sanguine, phlegmatic, choleric, and melancholic). In the Asian cultures, *Yellow Emperor's Canon of Medicine*, the premier book on medicine, makes reference to *Eum Yang 25 In* and *Oh Tae In* theories. All of these theories, however, were not based upon the functions of the internal organs. The first person to study and analyze the functions of the internal organs and propose the idea of *Chejil* was Dong Moo Yi Jae Ma in 1894 in his writing *Dong Eu Soo Sae Bo Won,* where he proposed *Sahsahng* medicine. *Sahsahng* medicine divides *Chejil* into four different categories: *Tae Yang In, Tae Eum In, Soh Yang In,* and *Soh Eum In*, depending upon the strength and weaknesses of the internal organs. At the Tokyo International Scientific Conference in 1965, Dr. Kwon Do Won further expanded *Chejil* into eight categories of *Keum Yang,*

Keum Eum, Mok Yang, Mok Eum, Toh Yang, Toh Eum, Soo Yang, and *Soo Eum*. In announcing his Eight *Chejil* Medicine, Dr. Kwon was able to incorporate both acupuncture and pulse diagnosis, two areas lacking in *Sahsahng* medicine.

Sahsahng Medicine

Sahsahng medicine was first introduced by Yi Jae Ma (1836-1900) in his book *Dong Eui Soo Seh Bo Won* written right after the *Chosun* era. He followed the Four Origin Constitution Theory and divided people according to their internal organs' strengths and weaknesses into four different *Chejils*—*Tae Yang In*, *Tae Eum In*, *Soh Yang In*, and *Soh Eum In*.

The difference between Yi's ideas and existing oriental medicine is that *Sahsahng* medicine is based on looking at the strengths and weaknesses of one's internal organs (i.e., *Chejil* medicine), while oriental medicine is based on the principles of the five elements of *Eum(-) Yang(+)*, thus putting the focus more on the symptoms and patterns of one's body. According to *Chejil* medicine, most diseases are caused by excessive imbalances between the internal organs of one's body. When the *Sahsahng* medicine theory was proposed in 1894, it was considered revolutionary among both eastern and western medicine.

Dr. Yi once said that one hundred years after his death, everyone would be able to understand this theory and that as it spreads throughout the world, "every household will be able to fix their own sicknesses and live long, healthy lives."

Originally a philosopher who later decided to study oriental medicine, Dr. Yi connected the two areas of his studies to come up with his theory. His decision to study oriental medicine was most likely due to his desire to treat his own sickness. Having been sick since he was a child, Yi realized that it was hard to diagnose his own sickness using traditional methods. His innate *Chejil* was the main problem, which led to the development of *Chejil* medicine. For example, when two people suffer from the same sickness, one may get better through treatment while the other does not, possibly getting worse or suffering side effects from the medication. Those who work in the medical field have probably dealt with this problem at least once in their career, wondering how the variety of responses to medication can possibly be made consistent.

Before *Sahsahng* medicine was founded by Dr. Yi, many other *Chejil* theories were discussed in both eastern and western medical fields. In *Nae Kyung*, the classic literature of oriental medicine, various theories such as *25 Human of Eum Yang, Five Forms of Human Theory, Jang Kyung Yak,* and *Eum Yang Human Theory* are included, while in western medical history, Hippocrates, known as the Father of Medicine, divided people into those who are plethoric, choleric, phlegmatic, and melancholic. Eppinger and Hess went on to divide people into those with sympathetic nerves and those with parasympathetic nerves. These theories, however, were not as helpful in describing how to appropriately treat patients according to the strengths and weaknesses of the internal organs. Therefore, these earlier theories did not accurately analyze people's health and the proper treatment needed to cure various sicknesses.

The driving principle of *Sahsahng* medicine, as well as Dr. Yi's purpose in creating this theory, is for people to know their individual *Chejils* in order to consume the types of food and live the kind of lifestyle that will help prevent sickness and promote health. When compared to traditional medical practice, in which a certain illness is thought to be caused by the same source, *Sahsahng* medicine is based on a much more fundamental and concrete foundation—a revolutionary achievement that merits praise.

As someone who consistently experiences the benefits of *Chejil* medicine, I would like to personally thank and give much respect to Dr. Yi and his outstanding work and accomplishments.

The Classification of *Sahsahng* Medicine

Tae Yang In

Tae Yang In refers to people with well-functioning lungs but a weak liver. People who fit this type have sharp eyes, are always in a hurry, are short-tempered, self-righteous, thoughtful, imaginative and creative, but do not socialize very well with others and are not very realistic. They are typically very thin with small hips and a weak lower body. Women within this classification typically have a hard time during pregnancy. They urinate very often and in large amounts. Less frequent urination in such a person would indicate a health problem. People who fit the *Tae Yang* in classification should eat more vegetables than meat; leaf vegetables are preferred over root vegetables.

Tae Eum In

Tae Eum In is the opposite of *Tae Yang In*, indicating a well-functioning liver but weak lungs. People who fit this type are usually very relaxed and not talkative. They have a high tendency to be obese and have thicker stomachs and waists. Their shoulders are weaker than their lower body. Though rare, slim *Tae Eum Ins* might occasionally be mistaken for *Soh Eum Ins*. They have kind personalities and are quite conservative, in that they do not like change. *Tae Eum Ins* are better off eating more meat than vegetables and need to eat root vegetables rather than leafy ones in order to be healthy. Some may get dizzy after taking medication for high blood pressure. Others will have a hard time digesting food, especially if they decide to eat large amounts of fruits and vegetables. *Tae Eum Ins* have warm bodies and tend to sweat a lot. Decreased perspiration would indicate a health problem.

Soh Yang In

Soh Yang Ins include people with well-functioning spleens but weak kidneys. They are usually short-tempered, extroverted, rigid, very chivalrous, affectionate, and quite sentimental. On the other hand, they get easily tired of things they have started and are not very good with bringing closure to tasks at hand. Their chest and shoulders are more developed than their lower body, meaning their body shape resembles that of an inverse triangle. Most are similar to *Tae Eum Ins* in that they can be larger in stature. Many *Soh Yang Ins* may tend to vomit bile if large amounts of bread, *dduk* (rice cake), or acidic fruits are consumed. More than half of diabetic patients fit in this group. A *Soh Yang In's* back may become easily injured if overworked, and headaches are common with an increase in blood pressure. Constipation would indicate poor health, and the persistence of this problem could lead to serious illness. Although *Soh Yang Ins* have good digestive systems, many suffer from gastroenteric troubles.

Soh Eum In

Soh Eum Ins are the opposite of *Soh Yang Ins* in that they have strong functioning kidneys but weak spleens. They are always very careful, delicate, tidy, and can be perfectionists. Their lower body is more developed than the upper body with a wide pelvis and big hips. They do not drink much water and tend to like warm things. Many do not feel any kind of discomfort even without going to the bathroom for 10 days. Many *Soh Eum Ins* have gastroptosis because of weak digestive systems and have a low body temperature, which is why they should eat lightly. Also, because they do not sweat much; profuse sweating would be an indicator of bad health.

8 *Chejil* (Constitutional) Medicine

At the Tokyo International Scientific Conference on October 24, 1965, Professor Kwon Do Won introduced the idea of the eight *chejils*, which included *mok yang, mok eum, keum yang, keum eum, soo yang, soo eum, toh yang,* and *toh eum.* He also proposed a new way that acupuncture and pulse diagnosis could appropriately be used—a notion unaddressed by the preceding *Sahsahng* theory.

In comparing eight *Chejil* medicine with *Sahsahng* medicine, a correlation exists between *Mok Yang/Mok Eum* and *Tae Eum Ins, Keum Yang/Keum Eum* and *Tae Yang Ins, Soo yang/Soo eum* and *Soh Eum Ins,* and *Toh Yang/Toe Eum* and *Soh Yang Ins,* respectively. Kwon Do Won, professor at Seoul National University's medical school and teacher of Dr. Lee Myung Bok, writer of *Know Your Chejil, Know Your Health,* has become an icon in the medical field. Professor Kim Yong Ok, once praised him, saying, "I have met two gods in my life. One was Mozart, and the other was Dr. Kwon Do Won." The following section describes the eight *Chejils,* as presented by Dr. Kwon.

Mok Yang Chejil

People who fall under the *Mok Yang Chejil* have good

functioning livers but weak lungs and are generally quite reserved. They tend to listen to people rather than talk, partially due to their weak lung capacity. They can tire easily with excessive talking. Singing may also be difficult because of their weaker lungs; many are tone deaf. They can get headaches or even go into shock if any glucose shots are administered to them. They are, however, quite resistant to anesthesia so it may take a while for it to take effect, and may wear out much faster than expected. They do not have any subjective symptoms even with an increase in blood pressure. Prescribing any blood pressure medication to such patients is difficult, as they may become weak and dizzy. *Mok Yang Ins* favor meat over fruit and any kind of acidic food.

Mok Eum Chejil

Mok Eum Chejil people have good functioning gall bladders but weak large intestines and are more outgoing than *Mok Yang Ins*. They usually have bowel movements numerous times a day—once between breakfast and lunch and again between lunch and dinner. In other words, they have good digestive systems, especially right after a meal. Their excrements are usually soft or watery like diarrhea, which is normal for them. This is because their short and weak large intestines are not able to handle the moisture very well, and since the water storage is so small, it needs to be excreted as often as possible. *Mok Eum Ins* are more short-tempered, sensitive, and emotional than *Mok Yang*

Ins. Many alcoholics are included in this group.

Keum Yang Chejil

Keum Yang Chejil people have good functioning lungs but bad livers and are short-tempered, arbitrary, and tend to get frustrated easily when things do not go their way. They are very firm, decisive, progressive, and extremely heroic and proud. They are also clear-headed, thoughtful, and are especially prone to atopic hypersensitivity and various allergies, especially in the nose area. Lumbago or stomach aches will occur as a sign of unhealthiness, while good urinating patterns indicate good health. They have a weak and thin lower body which gives them a higher probability of getting *hae yuk jeung*, a disease that makes the legs weak. In the case of females, they tend to have a hard time during pregnancy and childbirth and also experience excruciating pain during menstruation.

Keum Eum Chejil

Keum Eum Chejil people have well-functioning large intestines but bad gall bladders and are prone to rare diseases. If too much meat is consumed, they may have a higher risk of suffering from Parkinson's, Alzheimer's or other diseases that are caused by a lack of dopamine, which then makes their legs and arms tremble. Looking back at the mad cow disease epidemic in England, where the cows lost their balance out of nowhere and died, the crisis may have been caused by the mixing of sheep's intestines from Australia and cattle feed. This mixture was originally thought to cause the cattle to grow healthier and be better breeders. Cows are herbivores; feeding them meat caused their bodies to react quite negatively. Many factories that produced the cows' food closed down after finding out the cause of the disease. This may not have happened had people known about the eight *Chejil* medicine theory.

Soo Yang Chejil

Soo Yang Chejil people have good functioning kidneys but weak spleens and get constipated easily. Some may not want to go to the bathroom for up to 10 days and still feel no pain. This is, however, not a problem for their health. If they take any medicine that makes them feel less constipated, it can actually be damaging. Most *Soo Yang Ins* are quite the perfectionists and do not trust people easily.

Soo Eum Chejil

Soo Eum Chejil people have good functioning bladders but weak stomachs and are very susceptible to gastroptosis. They are born with a small stomach so if they overeat, the stomach will become weak and sag to the bottom. Therefore, they must eat in small amounts and chew slowly. Barley and pork are very dangerous for them.

Toh Yang Chejil

Toh Yang Chejil people have well-functioning spleens but weak kidneys and are very short-tempered—they talk before they think. They are, however, very sentimental, loyal, responsible, and have strong spirits of volunteering—most are soldiers, police officers, fire fighters, or volunteers. Even a very small rise in blood pressure is very harmful for them. When the temperature of their fecal matter becomes elevated, this can mean serious illness. About 70% of diabetes patients are in this group.

Toh Eum Chejil

Toh Eum Chejil people have well-functioning stomachs but weak bladders and are usually larger in stature than *Toh Yang Ins*. They have very well-developed shoulders and in a woman's case, large breasts. Most Japanese sumo wrestlers are probably in this group—they have large stomachs with especially strong digestive systems. A shot of penicillin may cause dangerous shocks to their bodies.

Distinguishing Your *Chejil*

Dr. Lee Myung Bok once said, "If you know your *Chejil*, you know your health." That's right. Knowing your own *Chejil* is the most important key for living a long and healthy life without sickness. Dr. Lee was not able to treat his own sickness, which he had for twenty to thirty years, but has since been fully cured with the help of professor Kwon Do Won's eight *Chejil* acupuncture treatments. Afterward, he learned Dr. Kwon's eight *Chejil* medicine and remains actively involved in the medical field even though he is now over 90 years old.

There are four important criteria in distinguishing *Chejil*—overall appearance (figure), personality (temperament), physiology, and pathology. A single thing, however, cannot easily determine one's self, which is why it is hard to distinguish *Chejil*. Many who have read anything about *Chejil* have probably dealt with the confusing thought of, "I think I'm a *XX In*... No wait, maybe I'm an *OO In*... I'm not quite sure..." Or perhaps there was an experience where one was diagnosed as a *Tae Eum In* at clinic A, but a *Soh Yang In* at clinic B, and then as a *Soh Eum In* at clinic C. Why all the different results? In reality, there is a limit to deciding one's *Chejil* if one's appearance and personality are the only factors taken into account. When looking at one's facial appearance, it would be wrong to simply compare it to someone else's face or to just look at a specific portion of it. Similarly, looking at one's physique, one cannot simply look at a specific section, but would have to make an overall comparison to make a fair assessment. However, many mistakes can be made by looking solely at one's physique or appearance since body forms may change through such external factors as exercise, sickness, or accidents. Personalities can also change due to different environments, education, religion, relationships, work places, experiences, and even through personal willpower. One might, for example, look a lot like one parent while having the same personality as the other; others can drastically change during their high school years through their friends; someone who was a major introvert can become an extreme extrovert after serving in the army; a generous single man can change into a stingy married husband, and so on. Therefore, it is hard to judge *Chejil* only through one's personality and appearance. Again, it is important to take all four criteria mentioned above into account, as well as the eight *Chejil* pulse diagnosis created by Dr. Kwon Do Won.

A mistake in this process can result in various sicknesses or even chronic diseases. How, then, can one be sure of one's *Chejil?* One is to take the appropriate acupuncture or oriental medicine and see how well the body responds to it.

One cannot be 100% sure just by looking at one's face, personality, or some sort of medical equipment. It is only through a customized series of acupuncture, medicine, and vitamins that will best confirm one's *Chejil.* Side effects to the treatment would indicate that one is of a different *Chejil* than previously thought. If, for example, one were diagnosed as a *Soh Yang In* and started to take the appropriate medications and food, such as Vitamin E, pork, barley rice, shellfish, watermelon, strawberries, and melon, but started getting stomach aches and diarrhea, that would indicate a misdiagnosis.

For several years now, many professionals have invested their time and money to find a more efficient way to distinguish one's *Chejil* using the eight *Chejil* medicine theory. Although various instruments were made for this purpose, no single one is able to precisely determine one's *Chejil*. Again, no one should expect 100% accuracy in this area.

I look forward to a *Chejil* diagnostic procedure in which one can use genetics to find out *Chejil*. If such a procedure gave 100% accurate results, I believe it would not only be worthy of a Nobel Prize, but it would be a very important and ground-breaking event in medical history and will be tremendously beneficial to society.

How to find your Chejil (Yes / No)

I sleep well when I have coffee or coke late afternoon or in the evening.

YES I gain weight easily
- **Y** Tae Eum In
- **N** So Eum In

NO I gain weight easily
- **Y** So Yang In
- **N** My lower body is larger than upper body
  - **Y** So Eum In
  - **N** Tae Yang In

I sleep well when I have coffee or coke late afternoon or in the evening.

YES I sweat normally
- **Y** Tae Eum In
- **N** So Eum In

NO I sweat normally
- **Y** So Yang In
- **N** I am meticulous and orderly.
  - **Y** So Eum In
  - **N** Tae Yang In

I am constipated often (I am not using any medicine.)

YES I don't feel uncomfortable even though I don't empty my bowel for 2~3 days.
- **Y** So Eum In
- **N** So Yang In

NO I gain weight easily
- **Y** Tae Eum In
- **N** My lower body is larger than upper body.
  - **Y** So Eum In
  - **N** Tae Yang In

I sweat normally.

YES I sleep well when I have coffee or coke late afternoon or in the evening.
- **Y** My shoulder is narrow.
  - **Y** Tae Eum In
  - **N** So Yang In
- **N** My excrement is wet and sometimes I have a bowel motion right after meal.
  - **Y** Tae Eum In
  - **N** So Eum In

NO My lower body is larger than upper body .
- **Y** So Eum In
- **N** Tae Yang In

*You may determine your Chejil to be the one with the most corresponding answers.
-The chart does not guarantee 100% accuracy-

II

Chejil and Food

|

"There is nothing in the mountains and fields that cannot be used as medicine"

Chejil and Food

The drama *Huh Joon* became a big hit when it aired awhile ago. Not only was it entertaining, but it also focused quite a bit on oriental medicine. In one particular scene there is an explanation of oriental medicine. Teacher Yoo Eui Tae says to his pupil Huh Joon, "Go to the mountains and fields and find something that cannot be used as medicine." Huh Joon then goes on his journey but comes back tired, restless, and empty-handed. When he comes back, his teacher asks him, "What have you brought back?" Huh Joon answers, "I'm sorry, teacher, but there was nothing I could find in the mountains and fields that fit your criteria." At this, teacher Yoo looks satisfied and responds, "You have learned well—there really is nothing in the mountains and fields that cannot be used as medicine." That is right. Everything in nature has its own unique medical characteristics. Anything that goes into the body, therefore, can be used as medicine. Many items used in oriental medicine can be easily found on a dining table. The difference between oriental medicine and regular food is that oriental medicine has been studied for hundreds of years in order to distinguish the foods that have large amounts of good medication. Regular food is also considered to have medical benefits, and such foods are the most practical and beneficial to everyday life. Many food items have the same effects as oriental medicine, which include items that cool down or heat up the body, help the lungs, liver, digestive system and kidneys, and strengthen the interior, exterior, spirit, and blood of the body. Internal organs are consistently and naturally unbalanced in relation to each other. To change that natural imbalance by eating something disagreeable to one's body type would not be healthy. For example, if a *Tae Eum In* starts eating food that makes the liver healthier instead of the lungs, the liver will get too strong, while the lungs get weaker, thus furthering the imbalance between the internal organs and ultimately damaging the body. Many of the patients I have had in the past made me realize how important food is to one's overall health. When I give my patients lists of food they should and should not eat according to their *Chejils*, most of them who have been struggling with a long period of sickness say, "There's nothing that I like on this list. What can I do when I'm not allowed to eat anything I like anymore?" This is the opposite for healthy people though. Their responses are, "I do not like anything that's on the 'should not' eat list anyway, so it won't be a problem for me." In other words, it was usually the people who ate things that were not fit for their *Chejils* that came in sick while people who ate things that were appropriate for their bodies were very healthy. This just tells us how important our everyday food is to our bodies and health. Food is like medicine. Eating what's right for one's *Chejil* is like taking the right kind of prescription pills, so know what's right for you!

The Good and the Bad

Tae Yang In

Good

A variety of Green vegetables, A variety of Fruits, Buckwheat, A variety of Fishes, A variety of Shellfishes, A variety of Green teas, Glucose, and Vitamin C

Bad

A variety of Meats, A variety of Dairy, Adlay, A variety of Nuts, A variety of Root vegetables, Ginseng, Coffee, Alcohol, Sunbathing, Sauna, and Vitamin A and D.

Tae Eum In

Good

A variety of Meats, A variety of Dairy, Adlay, A variety of Nuts, A variety of Beans(except Pinto Bean), A variety of Root vegetables, Coffee, Sunbathing, Sauna, and Vitamin A and D.

Bad

A variety of Green vegetable, A Variety of Fruits, Buckwheat, A variety of fishes, A variety of Shellfishes, A variety of Green teas, Wine, Glucose, and Vitamin C

Soh Yang In

Good

Pork, A variety of Fishes, A variety of Shellfishes, Eel, Catfish, Mudfish, Trout, A variety of Green Vegetables(except Wormwood, Allium Tuberosum), Aloe, A Variety of Squash, Barley, Mung Beans, Buckwheat, Cucumber, A variety of Melons, A variety of Berries, Banana, Pineapple, Egg white, Fish oil, Sunbathing, Sauna, and Vitamin E.

Bad

Chicken, Glutinous rice, Brown rice, A Variety of Beans, A variety of Nuts, Ginseng, Honey, Orange, Apple, Tangerine, Lemon, Lime, Tomato, Grapefruit, Seaweed, Kelp, Variety of Onions, Corn, Potato, Ginger, Wormwood, Allium Tuberosum, Curry, Black pepper, Mustard, Coffee, A variety of Vinegars, and Vitamin B and C.

Soh Eum In

Good

Chicken, Glutinous rice, Brown rice, Honey, Orange, Apple, Tangerine, Lemon, Lime, Tomato, Grapefruit, Seaweed, Kelp, Corn, Potato, Ginger, Wormwood, Allium Tuberosum, Curry, Black pepper, A variety of Vinegars, and Vitamin B and C.

Bad

Pork, A variety of Fishes, A variety of Shellfishes, Eel, Catfish, Mudfish, Trout, A variety of Green Vegetables(except Wormwood, Allium Tuberosum), Aloe, A Variety of Squash, Barley, Mung Beans, Buckwheat, A variety of Sweet Potatoes, Cucumber, A variety of Melons, A variety of Berries, Banana, Pineapple, Egg white, Excessive drinking of water, Beer, Coffee, Sunbathing, Sauna, Green teas, Fish oil, and Vitamin E.

*specific disease or diabetes can be exceptions.

*Foods not listed in The Good and The Bad need to be consumed in moderation. Had often or in large quantities can be harmful.

Too Much Fruit is Not Always Good

Last November, I had a chance to visit Korea with my wife. The cold frosty weather greeted us as we stepped out of the airport and refreshed our heads from the long flight. When we got to my sister-in-law's home, we unpacked our belongings and enjoyed a variety of fresh fruit along with tea. We caught up with each other and told many stories, and as the day went by, dinner came. I was somewhat worried when another round of fruit with tea was served right after dinner because both my father-in-law and sister-in-law are *Tae Eum Ins* like my wife, and for them, fruit and green tea were found on the "bad" list. I found some relief when my sister-in-law started talking about how she would get extremely dizzy and suffered from tinnitus (ringing in the ears). When I asked her for more details, she told me that she had dizzy spells and she would need to lie down as slowly as possible. Upon doing so, there were times when she could not even open her eyes because of her intense dizziness. The tinnitus was also severe, along with occasional migraines. As I told her that it was because of all the fruit she had been eating, she told me how ridiculous that was. "How can fruit give me dizziness, tinnitus, and migraines all at once?" she asked. I asked her what kind of fruit she ate regularly and how frequently. She answered that she ate an apple every morning and evening and also ate other types of fruits during the day. She probably ate more fruit than even rice. She then informed me that all the dizziness and tinnitus has been occurring for about a year. I asked if she had experienced the dizziness and tinnitus even before she had begun consuming so much fruit. She thought for a while and answered, "I think it was afterwards." I said, "You might think it's just a coincidence, but all that fruit you've been eating has actually amplified the imbalance among your internal organs, which has caused the dizziness and tinnitus." She still did not want to believe me, so I suggested that she give up fruit for a couple of days to see the result for herself. On the third day of her new diet, and accompanied by a specialized acupuncture treatment, she started to feel better. She was still doubtful that the fruit she was eating was the cause of her sickness. I addressed with her the common misconception that fruit is completely beneficial for everyone. The most of the victims of this misunderstanding are usually *Tae Eum Ins* and if they do not fix these thoughts, they will remain unhealthy. No matter how convincing and widely believed those theories are, they are worth nothing if more harm than good is done to the body.

Even though fruit is considered a healthy item, it only applies to those who have the appropriate *Chejil.* Many of the patients I have had are a lot like my sister-in-law—they decide to eat a lot of fruit because they have heard that it was good for their health and skin, might help them lose weight, or perhaps prevent diseases later in life. It should be known that fruit is not for everyone, and that there are certain fruits that are better for some than others, according to one's *Chejil*. Apples are good for *Soh Eum Ins* while watermelon, melons, strawberries, and bananas are good for *Soh Yang Ins*. *Tae Eum Ins* should eat only pears and apricots—all others may be bad for them. *Tae Yang Ins* are the only group who benefit from eating any kind of fruit.

The Side Effects of Various Fruit Juices

A good friend of mine once called worried because his son, who was in his twenties, had a hard time breathing, was always dizzy, and got frustrated for no apparent reason. When I saw him, I initially thought he was a *Soh Yang In* because of his short and stout physique. He told me that he could not sleep at night because he could not breathe well throughout the day. He found that he would get frustrated for no reason and could not do anything because he felt so dizzy, even from simply blinking. I proceeded to do some check ups on him, including a blood test, but found nothing—everything was normal. I did find out, however, that he was a *Mok Yang Chejil* (*Tae Eum In*) with a pulse rate of eighty beats per minute, which was significantly faster than normal, yet he had normal blood pressure. The reason for his dizziness and insomnia was due to a negative consumptive fever in his heart, which was caused by his daily intake of orange and cranberry juices that started about a month before his visit. The patient obviously had no idea that the fruit juices he had been drinking were harming his body. He was still confused when I told him that the juices made his stomach and heart heat up. I administered an acupuncture treatment that would cool down his stomach and heart—his chest and head instantly became very

43

clear and light. I told him not to drink any kind of fruit juice and to return the next day. Upon his return, he told me that all the stuffiness had cleared up by at least 50% and that he was able to sleep quite well. I gave him the same acupuncture treatment as before, prescribed him five days' worth of medication, and told him to come back after those five days. When he came back, he said that his sickness had gone away, and he had, in turn, been sleeping very soundly and was performing well at his workplace. After one last round of acupuncture, his illness was completely cured.

Because people in general think that fruit is very good for their health, they tend to eat fruit and drink its juices without any doubts. In addition, many people buy and take health and high nutrition fruit products without much thought. Therefore, it would be quite hard to believe that fruit can actually be bad to the body. But it is true—if one is not of the appropriate *Chejil*, fruit can really be damaging to the body. *Tae Eum Ins* will get a very bad stomach-ache if they decide to eat a lot of fruit. Of course, it would be healthy to eat certain fruits according to one's *Chejil*. *Soh Yang Ins* should eat watermelon, melons, strawberries, bananas, and pineapples, but stay away from apples, oranges, lemons, tomatoes, mangos, and tangerines (Refer to *The Good and the Bad* section). Remember, if you notice your health deteriorating due to consistent intake of any kind of fruit-based nutrition or health product, it might not be fit for your *Chejil*.

Can Green Tea Be Harmful?

A short and stout lady in her early forties came into my office saying that her body did not feel healthy. She had been having problems for the past five years with her legs, face, and hands, which would swell up constantly. She experienced weight gain and constipation, along with the feeling that something was stuck in the back of her throat, causing discomfort and coughing fits. She also felt congestion in her head when she woke up every morning. In addition, her right knee started to swell up and cause pain about two years before her visit. She was diagnosed to be a *Mok Eum Chejil* (*Tae Eum In*) and her pulse rate was about 85 beats per minute, which was quite fast. I administered the appropriate acupuncture treatment, gave her a list of what to eat, and what not to eat and told her to follow a diet according to that list. Starting the next day, she started taking herbal medication (*chung pae sa gan tang*), which I had prescribed, as well as more acupuncture. On the third day, she told me that the swelling had gone down and that her head and body felt much lighter. The coughing had gone away as well. On her fourth visit, however, she said that the swelling had returned. When I asked her if there was anything that she had been eating or drinking consistently since her last visit, she exclaimed, "That's it!" It was the green tea that she had been drinking for about five years, coinciding with the time that she started to feel sick. She told me that she had been regularly drinking five to ten cups of green tea daily for the past five years. When I asked her why she drank so much and for such a long time, she responded, "I read in newspapers and magazines that green tea helps you lose weight, prevents all kinds of diseases, including cancer, gives healthier skin, and makes you healthier in general. I just started drinking green tea instead of water." So I informed her that while green tea may be good for some that is not the case for *Tae Eum Ins* like herself. After ten days passed, she returned to my office saying that her knees felt lighter, the pain had gone away, and that her neck, head, and stomach felt a lot better than before. Her swelling disappeared, which was noticeable to those around her. She was very happy with the vast improvement in her health.

Whenever I meet patients like this, I always think and hope that *Chejil* medicine would become more widely known so that people would know their *Chejils* and know what to eat and what to stay away from, in order to live a long and healthy life.

For a while now, green tea has become widely known as a health product through newspapers and magazines. I do not doubt the benefits of green tea in cancer prevention, diabetes, and chronic fatigue. There are many kinds of vitamins and minerals in green tea that provide benefits to cells, in turn renewing the body and improving one's immune system. The green tea helps neutralize acidity in the body and helps many ailments such as constipation, high blood pressure, cholesterol, diarrhea, and headaches. It helps the skin and heart and aids in weight loss. However, *Tae Eum Ins* and *Soh Eum Ins* should not drink too much green tea because it can really be damaging, while *Tae Yang Ins* and *Soh Yang Ins* could benefit from drinking green tea.

Green Vegetables Can Be Poisonous

A heavy-set African-American woman in her mid sixties came to my office once with her 30-year-old son. He was a taxi driver around Los Angeles's Koreatown. She had recently come to the states from Ethiopia. He told me that she had serious migraines and that her whole body hurt so much that no one could even touch her. Her knees and ankles hurt especially, which made it difficult for her to walk and sleep. Her sickness had been around for thirty years and became practically unbearable. When I asked her son what kind of treatments his mother had received, he told me that every hospital she visited found nothing wrong. She was simply prescribed diuretics and steroids, along with some morphine. None of the treatments worked and her pain just got worse. She was about 160 cm (5'2") tall, weighed over 118 kg (260 pounds), and had swelling all over her body. I asked him for a list of her medications because I thought perhaps she had a serious addiction. Pain killers, blood pressure medication, and diuretics, however, were all that she took. Her pulse rate was very fast, at about 90 per minute, and was a *Mok Yang Chejil* (*Tae Eum In*). The first thought that crossed my mind was that she ate a lot of vegetables. My suspicions were correct—she had revealed that she had been eating many vegetables for the past thirty years. I was again saddened at the fact that she was a victim of modern medicine. I told her that her diet was what caused her sickness, but both she and her son did not seem to believe me. So I asked them whether they found it strange that she had been struggling with this sickness for over thirty years—roughly the same amount of time that she had been eating so many vegetables. At this, she and her son looked at each other quite confused. "How can vegetables and fruit damage my body like this?" I proceeded to describe to her what *Chejil* medicine is and told her that her diet should actually focus more around meat than vegetables and fruit. She found that extremely strange and I found it quite hard to convince the family, so I went ahead and suggested that we try the treatment and see what happens. I told her to eat only meat and root vegetables the opposite of what she had been eating. I finally convinced them to go home and try the regimen for at least two weeks. The next day, I gave her an acupuncture treatment that would neutralize the poisonous effect made by the green leafy vegetable she had previously consumed. She said that her knees, ankles, and head felt much lighter than before. In a good mood, she returned home and started taking the herbal medication I gave her (*chung pae sa gan tang*) while eating according to her prescribed diet plan. She lost eight pounds in a week and her pain started to go away so much that she could walk better. Three weeks after her treatment, she lost more weight, the headaches disappeared, and she could walk without pain. At the end of her treatment, I told her to keep eating as she had been and to call if any other problems arose.

Eating Meat
Can Lower Cholesterol (1)

I was curious to know how a close friend of mine, whom I had known ever since I first moved to LA, was doing. Surprisingly, he came into my office one day. I asked him how his health had been lately and found out he had undergone heart surgery due to a clog in the coronary artery. He then said that he was worried about his cholesterol level, as it had not dropped at all even after the surgery. Knowing his *Chejil* very well I said to him, "Of course your cholesterol level has remained the same." Seeing his surprised expression, I further inquired, "Did the hospital tell you not to eat meat because it can raise your cholesterol level and instead to eat only vegetables, fruit and fish?" "Yes, that's what I'm doing now," he said. "Why do you think your new diet isn't working?" I asked. "Well, that's what I'm here for…" was his solemn reply. His wife was and is currently a nutritionist at a major hospital in the US. So, you can already sense how strict she would have been about what he ate, especially after his surgery. No matter how hard they tried, however, his cholesterol level stayed the same. I told him to stay away from vegetables—leafy green ones in particular—and all fruits aside from pears. I further recommended that he increase his intake of meat while decreasing the amount of shellfish, sushi, and fish that he ate. He was very surprised and asked, "What kind of sham is that?" As a *Tae Eum In*, green leafy vegetables and fruit were harmful for him. He should have been eating root vegetables and meat in order to lower his cholesterol level." Though he probably questioned my sanity, I continued, "I know this is hard to believe in the current state of modern medicine, but there's a quote I like that says, 'results judge the value of theories.'" I believed then, as now, in the truth of this quote. No matter how persuasive a theory sounds, there's no use for it if it is not empirically proven. If my friend's cholesterol level was not going down even though he was only eating what was supposedly good for his cholesterol, couldn't there have been some sort of alternative? I told him to come back after he thought about what I had said. About a week later, he dropped by because he was in the area. I tried to further convince him that *Tae Eum Ins* have strong functioning livers but weak lungs, and that it was important to eat a lot of meat, not vegetables or fruit that can perhaps raise one's cholesterol level even more. We decided that we would let the results speak for themselves. We said our good byes and for the next few days, he called and visited a couple more times—it seemed like he was becoming more and more convinced of what I had been telling him. He said that he had a talk with his doctor and informed him of what I had been telling him. The doctor responded that maybe he should try out the treatment I suggested, as he had heard something about *Chejil* medicine in the past. He asked my friend to get the exact treatment method from me so that he could follow it thoroughly. I gave him the list of what to eat and what not to eat. About two months later, he gave me a call and exclaimed, "I just got my blood test results back and this is unbelievable!" He immediately rushed over to my office so that I could see the actual results. When I saw his copied results, his cholesterol level (LDL level) went down from 60 to 30 in just two months. Both he and his doctor were surprised at this. The drastic decrease happened because he had adjusted his diet according to his *Chejil* type.

Many of you probably think this is nonsense but these were the actual results that came from the hospital. The challenge is that modern medicine generally views meat as a raiser of cholesterol levels. *Tae Eum Ins*, though, especially need to be careful about this because their bodies work differently. My friend, who always liked meat, is now enjoying his new diet, which only consists of meat and never green leafy, fruit, shellfish, and shrimp, and is still very healthy.

Eating Meat
Can Lower Cholesterol (2)

Another good friend, whom I have known for about 20 years, came to visit me one day. He was suffering from frozen shoulders for two years and was wondering if there was anything I could do to help. He told me it hurt so much that it was hard for him to comfortably go the bathroom and even take a shower since his stiff shoulders would not let him lift his arms up. I explained to him the wonders of *Chejil* medicine while catching up on other stories and later found out that he was a *Mok Eum Chejil* (*Tae Eum In*). I then checked his arm mobility and gave him an appropriate acupuncture treatment. He was surprised to see that his arms functioned better right after the treatment. As I gave him his food list and told him he needed to come back for regular acupuncture treatments, he was shocked to see that green leafy vegetables were harmful to him. I told him it was wise for *Tae Eum Ins* to eat more meat rather than leafy vegetables and fruit and warned him to accurately follow the list that I had given him. In addition, he told me of other times when he felt uncomfortable after eating green leafy vegetables. At one point, he got rashes on his chest area, which would get better when he ate meat. The frozen shoulder he had was completely treated after 4 weeks and he was able to move his arms again.

After that incident, he called me again to talk about his high school-aged son this time. They found out through a check-up that his cholesterol level was quite high, so he told his wife about *Tae Eum Ins* having to eat a lot of meat in order to lower it. Since his wife did not seem to believe him, he told me that she and their son would come into my office soon. He wanted me to convince his wife that what he was saying was true since she would not believe him. That Saturday, my friend's wife came in with her son and asked me, "What do you mean that meat will lower his cholesterol level?" I explained the basis of *Chejil* medicine to her and how each *Chejil* had a different set of standards in terms of food consumption. She was still not convinced and asked again, "How is it that what you're saying is totally the opposite of what I'm used to hearing?" I merely told her that her son could follow my treatment and see the results afterwards. "After all, results judge the value of theories, right?" She agreed, and as we went on about what he should eat, I stressed the importance of being very accurate with what her son ate. Even when eating a hamburger, he would have to take out the lettuce, tomatoes and pickles in order to follow the diet. Three months later she called to say that the blood test results had come in and that both she and her doctor were shocked. She sent me a copy of the results along with a testimonial letter highlighting her son's dramatic results. Needless to say, she was quite ecstatic. I heard recently from my friend that his son has been living a healthy life and has been sticking to his special diet of eating only meat and no vegetables.

The Harmfulness of Beans for *Soh Yang Ins*

While my wife and I were relaxing at home after a long day of work, the phone rang. My wife went to answer it because it is almost always for her. I heard her say, "How do you do, deaconess?" and knew at once it was one of the deaconesses from church wanting to talk to my wife. She surprisingly gave the phone to me, and when I answered, I found out that she used to be one of my patients. She told me her insides ached and that she had been vomiting stomach acid for about a month. She went to the hospital, where she was told she had hyperacidity along with stomach inflammation. She took the medication that had been prescribed to her, but her condition was not improving, hence her phone call to me. Since I knew her *Chejil*, the first thing I asked was if she had been taking any nutrition products that contained beans. She affirmed that she had—just as I suspected. Because beans have warm medical properties and help digestion, *Soh Yang Ins,* who already have strong and warm digestive systems will only get warmer by eating beans, thus amplifying the imbalance between the internal organs. Without treatment, this heat in the stomach causes hyperacidity. More drastically, the acid may backflow and cause inflammation and a gastric stomach. I suggested that she stop taking the products and see what happens. If the sickness did not go away, she was to get back to me as soon as possible. After a week had passed, I got curious so I gave her a call. She told me that all the stomach pain had disappeared. If she did not know about the bean product and kept on taking it, her health could have really been damaged. The reason why the medication prescribed by the hospital did not work was because it worked just like the beans. This is what I emphasize the most during treatments—the reason modern treatment often does not work is because there are so many different health and nutrition products that are being wrongly prescribed or misused.

Who would have thought that beans could cause such a health problem? People frequently say that beans are "field-grown meat" because it contains so much protein and fat. It can also be useful in many ways, such as with cancer prevention, diabetes, arthritis, lowering cholesterol levels, aging, and constipation. No matter how good it may seem, it can be harmful for *Soh Yang Ins*. They should therefore stay away from anything made of beans. If you eat *kong gook su* (cold bean noodles), soy milk, or rice with beans, only to experience a sour stomach, this would indicate that you are a *Soh Yang In*.

Chejil and Grain Rice

What kind of grain is good for one's health? This is the question many people ask because of the common thought that regular white rice is not nutritious enough. Some think that too much white rice can cause high blood pressure, diabetes, and paralysis, among other things. So, then, many try to mix white rice with various grains to provide more nutrients. Newspapers, magazines, and even TV shows preach that this or that grain is good for the body. Before we know it, we start mixing several different types of grain into our rice. This, however, just makes eating very uncomfortable. People say things such as, "If you want to treat constipation, eat brown rice," or, "You need to eat barley to help with diabetes," and so on. Of course they suggest this after they try it out and get good results. Not everyone experiences the same results, however. Rather, some might experience gas with the consumption of barley, or may vomit after eating brown rice. They complain how mixing grains gave them a hard time. This is because rice and all other kinds of grains have distinct characteristics that affect people in different ways. Many people, for example, eat brown rice because it supposedly prevents constipation and geriatric diseases. Many of them will vomit bile and get constipated instead, which means they're usually *Soh*

Yang Ins. If the results do come out positively, however, this probably means they are a *Soh Eum In.*

Another example concerns beans and the various health products made from it. Many of those who take these products actually become healthier but there are others who encounter digestive problems, bilious vomit, and gas or diarrhea. Such people are mostly *Soh Yang Ins* or *Tae Yang Ins* and the people who get good results are usually *Tae Eum Ins.* Another example is glutinous rice: Only *Soh Eum Ins* can get chronic stomachaches and constipation relieved through *dduk* (rice cakes) made from glutinous rice. If *Soh Yang Ins* try to do the same thing, however, it gives them an opposite effect by making the stomachaches worse. For them, barley is the better choice. I have treated serious stomachaches, constipation, headaches, skin disease, various allergies, and even high blood pressure for *Soh Yang Ins* just by telling them to eat barley. I hope that from now on, people will know what kind of grain to eat according to their *Chejils.* It is healthier to eat regular white rice than to force one to eat grain rice and possibly get sick. So how did rice, of all things, become a staple food in Korea? Perhaps it was because rice, out of any other grain, had the least side effects when given to various people. Whenever I go out to eat, some places make grain rice ready for people who want it instead of white rice. This is when I wish they would prepare various kinds of grain rice according to the different *Chejils.* A day may come where everything will be divided up according to this theory—the rice, side dishes, dessert, and even water. This is what I call the *Chejil* revolution and eating the right kind of grains would only be a small part of it.

Barley

In the 1960s, the Korean government promoted mixing flour based foods or barley into various foods due to a shortage in rice production. Since barley was good for the digestive system and health, the government wanted people to eat a lot of it and even set up an ideal ratio of rice to barley so people could refer to it whenever they made rice. Even in schools, teachers would check each student's lunches and see how much barley they had in their rice. If they did not have enough, they would strongly recommend students to bring more barley next time. Out of all grains, barley has the coldest medicinal properties, so it is an ideal product for the summer months when people usually eat barley rice in cold water or mixed with various things like *yul moo kimchi*, red chili paste, bean paste, or sesame oil. Barley contains a starch enzyme called diastase which helps the digestive system and also has much more fiber than regular rice. It has been known to lower cholesterol levels and prevent constipation by helping the large intestine do its job. It also lowers blood pressure for diabetes patients who are usually *Soh Yang Ins*. Because barley is so popular in terms of health, many families make barley tea and try to drink it instead of water. If barley is not right for your *Chejil*, however, it can be poisonous to your body. You probably know people who do not like to eat barley because they get stomachaches and diarrhea—they are usually *Soh Eum Ins* with weak digestive systems. Many pediatricians recommend that kids with colds or tonsillitis drink barley tea. This is because barley, with its cold medicinal nature will have a neutralizing effect on the body. If any *Soh Eum In* kids follow this, they can get sicker with symptoms such as higher fever and stomach aches. In such cases, they would need to stop drinking the tea immediately. On the other hand, the consumption of barley tea would definitely help *Soh Yang In* kids because barley suits their *Chejil*. We commonly see parents feeding baby formula containing barley to their infants to relieve any constipation. If any infant suffers any side effects, it undeniably would mean the child is a *Soh Eum In*. A patient of mine once asked for help saying that her one-year-old daughter had been suffering from excessive constipation so I told her to give me a list of food that she has been feeding her child. One thing that caught my eye was barley tea, so I suggested she stop feeding the tea at once and to call me after a few days. A week later, she came in to my office and happily informed me that her daughter's constipation had disappeared. I gave her a list of foods she should be feeding her daughter in order to prevent future constipation. The baby was definitely a *Soh Eum In*, just like her father who got treated for hip-gout.

Barley can be poisonous to *Soh Eum Ins* but it is the best medicine for *Soh Yang Ins* who have good digestion systems and a lot of body heat. It can heal their chronic gastro enteric troubles, headaches, diabetes, neuralgia, molars, chronic tiredness, and skin and other diseases, so it is good for them to drink barley tea instead of other drinks on a regular basis.

A friend of mine currently living in Philadelphia is a *Soh Yang In* who solved all of his digestive problems by simply drinking barley tea. When I visited him recently, he was still healthy and drinking the tea everywhere he went, even in his car.

Barley tea can easily be made by mixing barley and water and heating it up for an hour or so until the color turns pinkish. It can be served hot or can be stored in the refrigerator and consumed in place of water. But, this should be done only by *Soh Yang Ins*.

Soh Yang Ins and Brown Rice

Brown rice is very popular among many families nowadays because it is thought to be healthy. Many products like bread, tea, *dduk* (rice cake), and oil are made from it and can be easily found. It is especially known to treat geriatric diseases and is praised by many professionals, doctors, newspapers, magazines, and even TV programs.

Many housewives who hear this tend to go overboard by eating brown rice constantly, regardless of how much the family complains about its taste and texture.

Compared to white rice, brown rice contains many more nutrients and is thought to warm the spleen and stomach, thus speeding up digestion. Like any other grains, however, these effects do not apply to everyone. Only those with the proper *Chejil* can benefit from brown rice.

Soh Eum Ins are fit to eat brown rice while *Soh Yang Ins* are not. This is because *Soh Yang Ins* already have good digestive systems. By eating brown rice, the imbalance between the organs becomes greater, thus making them more prone to various diseases.

If a patient is taking the proper medication but a particular sickness does not seem to go away, it is important to see what kind of rice, food, nutrition, and health products are being consumed by the patient, and what kind of lifestyle he or she is living. Most likely, that patient is eating the wrong things and not living the life style he or she should be leading.

One day, a senile lady who just turned seventy came into my office saying that she had excessive abdominal pain. She explained how her stomach often got bloated and constipated, and that she had also been vomiting up bile and experiencing nausea. After coming home from the hospital, where she was told that she had inflammation of the stomach, she started to eat only soft and mild foods. The pain went away at first but soon came back, hence her visit to me. I diagnosed her as a *Soh Yang Chejil* (*Soh Yang In*) and found out that she had a lot of heat in the weak spots of the body. I initially gave her an acupuncture treatment, after which she told me her insides felt much better afterwards. As we talked more, I learned that she has been eating a lot of brown rice for awhile, and I determined that that was the main problem for her sickness. I suggested that she eat barley instead of brown rice and explained the relationship between brown rice and *Soh Yang Ins*. She came back the next day saying that her bloating and other pains had gone away. I prescribed her some medication and administered more acupuncture treatments and gave her a list of food she should be eating. She came back again after five months with the same problems. It turned out that she could not stop herself from eating brown rice because of its popularity, so I had to give her the same treatments as before and warned her numerous times that if she kept on with her bad habit, her health would seriously deteriorate.

III

Chejil
and
Nutrition Products

"Outcome Determines the Validity of the Theory"

Tae Eum Ins and Royal Jelly (A)

Mr. Kim, a former patient of mine in the sewing business, called one day worried about his mother. She was in her early seventies and could not get rid of her excessive headaches and high blood pressure no matter how much she took her medication. I asked if she had been taking any kind of nutritional products. He said that she had been taking royal jelly for about 5 days before the onset of pain. Although I have never met her, I knew that her son was a *Tae Eum In*, so I asked him, "You're a lot like your mother, aren't you?" He was surprised, and asked, "How did you know?" I told him that royal jelly is not good for *Tae Eum Ins* because they tend to experience a lot of side effects, like heavy headaches and higher blood pressure, just like my friend's mother.

A few days later, Mr. Kim came into my office with his mother. Her blood pressure was 200/100, so I gave her an acupuncture treatment. Afterward she said her head felt lighter. I told her to stop taking the royal jelly and to come back for a few more treatments. Three days later, her blood pressure level started to go down a little and after a full week, it went back to normal and her headaches were gone.

Tae Eum Ins and Royal Jelly (B)

There is a good *suhl lung tang* (beef soup) restaurant that I often go with a friend. On my last visit, the restaurant owner told me that he had been having headaches for a while and that they wouldn't go away. Since I knew she was a *Tae Eum In*, I asked her if she had been taking any of the following: Vitamin C, honey, royal jelly, green vegetable juice, fruit, or fruit juice. These were popular health products that are not beneficial for *Tae Eum Ins*. It turned out that she had started taking royal jelly right before the headaches started. I advised to stop taking them because that was what was causing the headaches. I also suggested that she get her blood pressure checked. Since she did not have a blood pressure monitor, she came to my office one afternoon. Her blood pressure turned out to be 190/100. I gave her an acupuncture treatment that would properly balance her internal organs, thus relieving the headaches. When I went back to eat at her restaurant a few days later, she welcomed me and let me know that her headaches had gone away and her blood pressure had gone down as soon as she stopped taking the royal jelly.

Royal jelly is a good nutrition product for *Soh Eum Ins*. It will take care of chronic headaches and strengthen the immune system, which can help prevent various diseases. *Tae Eum Ins* and *Soh Yang Ins*, however, do not benefit from the jelly.

Soh Eum In's—Side Effects of Nutritional Products

A wife of an old friend came into my office one day. I had seen her frequently in the past, but it had been a while. She had heard my interview on the radio and felt that she could benefit from the *Chejil* theory she had heard about. She heard in my interview of the side effects of various vitamins and nutritional products. I remember saying during the interview that there are so many different kinds of health products including various vitamins, minerals, and dietary supplements that too many people tend to take without thinking about any possible side effects. No matter how healthy the products sound, one can get sick from them if one is not of the appropriate *Chejil* for that product. I further stated that anyone experiencing ill effects from such products should go to the nearest clinic for oriental medicine. The reason for the danger in taking a large amount of health products is that out of so many of them, only about 3 are actually suitable for one's *Chejil,* while the other countless ones will be harmful. Thus, the probability for people taking the wrong product is much greater than not, and taking the wrong products may end tragically.

As a consequence, many patients that come into my office experience pain because of the misuse of health products. Instead of stopping the use of such products, they decide to continue on because they do not think the side effects are coming from products that are supposedly good for them.

So, I will say it again: If you or anyone you know is taking any kind of vitamins or nutrition and health products, even ones that are said to be naturally made, but seem to be suffering from side effects such as tiredness, various diseases, and constant weariness, quit using the products at once!

In addition, one may experience uneasiness, tiredness, and insomnia after quitting even though one's health may improve. The experience may be similar to withdrawal from cigarettes, alcohol, or drugs, so one must be mindful and endure such symptoms in order to be completely cured.

My friend's wife, mentioned above, showed symptoms such as restlessness, indigestion, headaches, dizziness, and stuffiness in the chest area. She had been taking multi-vitamins, vitamins E and C, calcium, glucosamine, an unidentified eye nutrition product, and fish oil. She felt the need to visit me because she was also experiencing the side effects I had described in my interview and wanted to know what was acceptable for her *Chejil*.

She turned out to be a *Soh Eum In*. After receiving the appropriate acupuncture treatment, she immediately felt her head get clearer and her insides more comfortable. I told her to stop taking the multi-vitamins, which isn't much use to anybody, as well as the vitamin E, fish oil, and the eye nutrition product. I told her to take vitamin B instead, since it's very effective for *Soh Eum Ins*. With that, I told her to come back the next day. When she did, she was quite amazed at how much her body changed—70% of the pain disappeared. After her second acupuncture treatment, she felt much better, and after four days, she was completely cured.

Vitamin E:
Harmful for *Soh Eum Ins*

While having lunch with a couple of friends, one of them commented that his back had been hurting and that it was getting worse. He had never had this problem before and didn't know what to do. He had never experienced a back injury and told me that one morning he got up from his bed and it just started to ache. When I asked if he had been taking any health products, he told me his wife suggested he take some vitamin E for his health. I knew at once that that was the problem, so I told him to stop taking it immediately. My other friends looked at me with suspicion, so I explained that he was a *Soh Eum In* (I could tell just by his appearance), which meant that he had innately good kidneys. By taking vitamin E, the imbalance between his organs intensified, causing the lumbago. Then I told the "patient" that since his wife is a *Soh Yang In*, she should be the one taking the vitamin E and that vitamin B would be better for him and his back pain. When I asked him about his back a few days later, he told me that the pain had disappeared like magic once he stopped taking the vitamin E.

When vitamins were first introduced to the world in the 1960s, it was a revolutionary event. I remember everywhere I went, vitamins were the hot topic.

Vitamins are organic substances, meaning there is

nothing to taking too much of it. Early on, people claimed that in the "future," taking vitamin pills a few times daily would substitute for any kind of solid food. Forty years have passed now and we are not even close to living off of vitamin pills. Instead, side effects are becoming more and more evident. Vitamin researchers and developers made the natural herbal vitamin, which were supposed to get rid of the side effects, but it did not work out as planned. The problem was and is that people do not realize that the side effects are solely due to the vitamins themselves. No matter how much I try to explain, many still think that it is impossible for vitamins to be bad for the body.

Many of the patients who come into my office say things like, "Because I was tired," "I was worried about my health," "Because everybody else was taking it," or "I felt that I should take it," when I ask them why they started taking vitamins. At first their bodies feel lighter and the tiredness seems to go away for a bit, but as time goes by, they start feeling sick and more tired than before. When this happens, they start talking to professionals, read health columns in newspapers or magazines, and decide to take more health products in addition to what they are already taking. This could lead to taking up to ten different products a day without even knowing the benefits or damage they do to the body. People who take so many of these products tend to get sick more often than people who are not taking anything at all.

The side effects include chronic tiredness, headaches, indigestion, skin disease, face discoloration, and swelling of the body. Of course, vitamins are essential and important nutrients that we all need. However, we need to take the right kind of vitamins in accordance with our *Chejils* if we do not want to experience negative side effects.

Vitamins and Skin Disease

A woman in her early fifties came into my office complaining how she could not wear short-sleeved shirts because of a skin infection on her left arm that occurred about five years ago. She also suffered from constant tiredness and migraines. When she went to the hospital, they could not figure out what was wrong and gave her some allergy medication, which did not help at all. As soon as I heard that, I knew her ailment had something to do with health products of some kind. Usually, when an illness cannot be explained by looking at test results, it is almost always due to products that are consumed but do not fit one's *Chejil*. The side effects get worse according to the amounts taken. I asked her if she was taking any nutritional products and she told me that she was. She was quite hesitant when I asked her to list the products she had been taking, and I was amazed at her answer. The amount of health products she owned and used was comparable to a neighborhood health product store. Her knowledge about those products was almost like that of a professional, and the amount she was taking daily was just unbelievable.

She and her husband would get up each morning and determine the best products that they thought were most needed for that day. These products came out to something between five and ten pills per day. They would do the same routine after they work to regain and boost their health. I tried my best to hide the amazement at this and asked whether they took all of these products to keep themselves healthy. She started explaining to me the importance of each of the vitamins and minerals she had taken and confidently said that she was in good health.

It seemed quite impossible to try to convince someone who almost religiously took heath products and knew about each and every one of them like a professional. I told her that while it is true that people need nutrients, the particular kind of nutrients needed for each *Chejil* are all very different. If she took products that she did not need as much, the imbalance between the internal organs would increase, thus causing various diseases and sicknesses. The problem is that people do not realize that what they're eating can actually be what's harming them. The woman's skin rash was an example of the side effects that can be caused by health products when taking too many of the wrong kinds. She gave me a very suspicious look so I kept on going, telling her to think about the time frame of when the rash first started and when she began eating all those vitamins and minerals. After a while, she replied that, indeed, she hadn't had any skin infections or the tiredness before she started taking the supplements. She was still not convinced though—she had too much knowledge about the products from the point of view of modern medicine. Since *Chejil* medicine was something so different, she would not easily buy it. As I had been telling so many of my patients, I said,

"Let's just try quitting the health products for two weeks and get some treatments started. We'll see what happens at the end of the two weeks." She agreed, and we started the treatment right away. I diagnosed her as a *Keum Yang Chejil* (*Tae Yang In*), and I remembered that almost none of the health products nowadays were suitable for this *Chejil*. That was why the side effects were much worse for her than for her husband. I gave her an acupuncture treatment that would neutralize the pains caused by the vitamins and told her to come back the next day. When she came back, she told me the headaches and the itchiness went down and her body felt much lighter. When I was certain that she was a *Keum Yang Chejil* (*Tae Yang In*) according to the treatment results, I gave her a list of foods she should and should not eat and told her to follow it very carefully. Ten treatments later, she was completely cured and amazed at how accurate *Chejil* medicine was and promised to come back with her husband next time.

Chejil and Calcium

Calcium is one of the five major nutrients we need, along with protein, fat, carbohydrates, and vitamins, and takes up over 90% of all inorganic elements in our bodies. Along with phosphoric acid, calcium is what the bones and teeth are made of, meaning that if we do not have enough, it can cause osteoporosis or stunt growth in children. Pregnant woman especially need to have enough calcium because without it, their bones can weaken, which can in turn have harmful effects on the fetus. Females will get stronger bones and can even lose weight with the right amount of calcium. It is also important in preventing osteoporosis for the elderly.

Some can get indigestion and tiredness by taking too much of it. This is because they have been taking forms of calcium not suitable for their *Chejil*. "What does this mean?" you might ask. Well, let's talk about what kind of calcium is good for your *Chejil*.

Not all calcium is the same but is dependent on its composition. Thus, calcium from cow bones or milk; shellfish and other kinds of sea food; seaweed and other marine plants; and coral are all different. *Tae Eum Ins* should get calcium from cow bones or milk, *Tae Yang Ins* from various seafood, *Soh Yang Ins* from cow bones or milk, coral, and seafood, and *Soh Eum Ins* from various marine plants such as kelp and seaweed. Doing this can greatly reduce the probability of experiencing any side effects. If you are using calcium and are experiencing indigestion, tiredness, headaches, or maybe even swelling, you should consider changing the type of calcium you are taking.

In April of 2002, an article entitled "Too Much Vitamin C Can Damage the DNA of White Blood Cells" was published in the health column of a certain magazine. "The period of eating Vitamin C like a snack is now over. According to a recent report from England, eating too much Vitamin C can increase the anti-oxidation level but can also damage the DNA of white blood cells, which is important for the immune system—*Seoul Central Hospital* (Sister hospital of Harvard Medical School)." *Tae Eum Ins* and *Soh Yang Ins* were applicable to this news.

Why might reports like this, on the side effects of vitamins, be published in this day and age? It is because of *Chejil*. Many think there is no relationship between vitamins and *Chejil*, but taking the right kinds of vitamins can easily prevent the occurrence of side effects. Most people start off with multi-vitamins, and when they hear that vitamin E is helpful in preventing aging, they add that onto the list. Next, they also hear that vitamin C is best in relieving tiredness and that vitamin B is excellent for anemia. In the end, one can end up taking up to ten different kinds of vitamins. Of course vitamins are a vital part of our lives, but it is only useful if it fits our *Chejil*. For example, vitamin E, which prevents aging, will strengthen kidneys, which means that *Soh Eum Ins* who already have strong kidneys and take vitamin E will get various side effects due to the amplified imbalance within the body if they take it. This vitamin is therefore particularly helpful for people who have weak kidneys—*Soh Yang Ins* to be specific. *Soh Eum Ins* need to take vitamin B to strengthen the stronger digestive system and *Tae Eum Ins* should take Vitamins A and D.

I emphasize again how important it is to take the appropriate vitamins and calcium according to our *Chejils* in order to get the results we want.

Chlorella

Every time a new health product comes out, it usually catches my attention right away because it can be either helpful or harmful depending on who takes it. Plus, there are some products containing elements that are both good and bad for each *Chejil*, which then would not help anyone at all.

The side effects that can occur through the misuse of a product can be chronic tiredness, indigestion, stomach-aches, abdominal pain, diarrhea, headaches, dizziness, itchiness, and even skin infection. The problem is that people do not realize all this comes from taking nutritional products. So, whenever a new product comes out, I worry that it will be good for some *Chejils* but dangerous for others. One of those is chlorella, a very popular product nowadays.

Chlorella was first found by a scholar named Beijerinck from the Netherlands and is also known as the "dream health product." It is made from green algae and contains a lot of chlorophyll and is more than 50% vegetable protein, which is more protein than what the "field meat" beans contain. It can be quite helpful for growing kids and weak senior citizens. It also contains not only vitamins and various minerals but also the eight essential amino acids as well as the necessary iron to produce red blood cells. The five essentials plus the forty or more nutrients that make up chlorella is highly alkaline which can neutralize acidity in one's body, thus strengthening the immune system. It is recommended in treating liver disease, diabetes, atopy hypersensitivity, osteoporosis, and constipation. It is also known to have chemotherapeutic effects and help the skin—it is indeed the medicine for everything. However, this product is only good for *Soh Yang Ins* and *Tae Yang Ins* and can be quite harmful for *Soh Eum Ins* and *Tae Eum Ins*.

One example is when a woman in her mid-forties came into my office saying that she had been suffering from indigestion, stomach and head aches, and dizziness for the past two months. She was diagnosed with gastric stomach about a month ago and told me although she has always had indigestion, her stomach never hurt this much before.

She was a *Soo Eum Chejil* (*Soh Eum In*) and experienced frequent chills. During the check up, I found out that she had started taking chlorella three months prior. Chlorella is harmful for *Soh Eum Ins*, which is why it felt so sick, so I told her to stop taking the chlorella immediately. I then gave her acupuncture treatments, informed her to come back the next day, and gave her five days' worth of medication. When she came back the following day, she said that her stomach felt a lot better and her dizziness went away as well. Two weeks later, she was completely cured.

Another patient in his early-fifties came in complaining about abdominal pains and headaches which was all due to the chlorella that he had been taking for about a month. He was a *Mok Eum Chejil* (*Tae Eum In*), and after a week of treatments and stopping the intake of chlorella, he was cured as well. As you can see, even a "dream product" can cause serious side effects.

Diabetes and Health Products

A man in his early-sixties came to my office one day. It turned out he had diabetes for 15 years, and no matter how much he took his diabetes medication (three times a day), his blood sugar level would not go down. In the mornings it would come out to be 200 and two hours after each meal, it would rise up to 300. Doctors recommended insulin treatments for him.

He was a *Toh Yang Chejil* (*Soh Yang In*), had a lot of deficient heat, and had a very fast pulse at ninety beats per minute. When I asked about his dietary habits, he said he had been trying not to eat anything harmful for diabetes and had been taking eight different kinds of health products, including multi-vitamins. I was certain that one of the products he had been taking must be the problem for his constantly high blood sugar level, so I told him to tell me all the things he had been taking. Out of the eight, vitamin E was the only acceptable one for *Soh Yang Ins* while the others were very harmful. When I told him this, he was surprised and said that a professional had recommended that he take these products since it would help with his diabetes. In reply, I informed him that vitamins C and B and ginseng were not helpful for *Soh Yang Ins* who already have good digestive systems, and since multi-vitamins contain vitamins

B and C, it was obviously not good for him. He was still confused as to why I did not want him to take the health products, so I told him we could discuss that after the treatments. I advised him to stop taking everything except for the vitamin E for a week and that we would check his blood sugar level on the next visit. We would then see who was right or wrong.

A week did not even pass when he came back saying that his blood sugar level went down to 125, which was around the normal level. I explained to him as I quoted again, "Results judge the value of theories. Don't you think that's true?" No matter how much a theory seems acceptable, it's useless if the treatments do not work. He agreed but was worried that he became restless, tired, sleepless, and frustrated even though his blood sugar level was back to normal now. I informed him that he was experiencing withdrawal symptoms since he had suddenly quit taking all those vitamins and health products. I told him the symptoms would go away in about a month, and then he'd be cured. I told him for future reference, to not take things just because people say it's good for you, and if he did try a new product, to be sure to check his sugar level every now and then. An increase in the level would indicate that he should immediately stop taking that product.

Vitamin C is Poison for Diabetes Patients (1)

For diabetes patients, measuring one's blood sugar level two hours after each meal is just as important as taking it every morning. While the morning blood sugar level might be in the normal range, diabetic patients can still experience arm and leg pains, vision trouble, and chronic tiredness two hours after meals. Many patients are relieved when blood sugar levels are within the normal range in the morning, but they really should be more careful with monitoring levels after meals.

When experiencing various side effects, a lot of these patients do not realize that it is because of their diabetes. When they check their blood sugar level at that point, it is usually very high. While the kinds of food they ate can be the reason for this, it is mostly the vitamins and health products they are taking (without taking into consideration their *Chejil*) that may be causing the sudden increase in blood sugar.

A patient of mine is a medical professional in his mid-fifties and has diabetes. He said that even though he was taking his diabetes medication and his blood sugar level was normal in the mornings, it always rose to 300 two hours after his meals and remained at that level. Since he was working in the medical field, I asked him if he had been taking vitamin C. As I had thought, he did not seem to be aware of the relationship between the vitamin C he was taking and his fluctuating blood sugar level. I told him that many vitamins could be harmful if they are not suited for one's *Chejil* and that vitamin C was one of those things harmful to his *Chejil*. Vitamin C could cause the blood sugar level to rise by 90% for all diabetes patients and according to my statistics, it's probably the main cause of diabetes. I then wanted to know if he had been taking any other kinds of products. He was confused, thinking vitamin C was required for the immune system, blood vessels, and blood circulation, especially among diabetics. I figured it would take a while to convince him about *Chejil* medicine since he had been a believer of modern medicine for a long time, so I just suggested that we try out my treatment first. I told him to stop taking the vitamin C and anything that contains it for a week and check his blood sugar level. If he saw the results, he would know whose theory is correct. In my experience, many people, especially *Soh Yang Ins*, started taking vitamin C right before they got diagnosed with diabetes. I asked him to give it one week. Although he was still skeptical about it, he agreed to follow my instructions and went home.

A few days later, he gave me a call reporting that his blood sugar level had gone back to normal after he quit taking the vitamin C. With satisfaction, I explained to him that this was only a small part of the unsolved mysteries in modern medicine that I believe can be solved with *Chejil* medicine, along with other treatments. No matter how convincing and logical a theory sounds, it is useless if it cannot be applied and proven in the real world. The truth is that only "results can judge the value of theories." As in this case, many of the facts we know about diabetes are incorrect and vitamin C is only a very small portion of it.

Vitamin C is Poison
for Diabetes (2)

A pastor in his early-sixties visited me through an old patient's referral. His face was quite dark and the coloration did not look so good. As it turns out, he was suffering from extreme diabetes, taking his diabetes medication three times a day along with 90 units of insulin. Even after four months of treatment, his blood sugar level in the mornings would be around 200-250, and after meals, it would rise to 350. Since it used to be in the 500s, he was satisfied with this. However, I wanted to know what was causing his elevated blood sugar level, so while consulting him, I found out he had been taking vitamin C as well as other vitamins right before his symptoms materialized. I told him to stop taking the vitamins right away. He had a shocked expression while his wife angrily asked what kind of doctor would suggest such a thing. I had to calmly explain that he was a *Soh Yang In* (*Toh Yang Chejil*) and that vitamin C is very harmful for both his *Chejil* and diabetes. It could have been the cause of his sickness, actually. I informed him that in order for him to stop taking the medication and insulin, and to get his blood sugar level back to normal, he needed to stop taking the vitamins. Since they still did not seem to believe me, I told him to try it out for a week, and then we could talk about the results afterwards. They skeptically agreed and went home. A few days later, they told me that they had to start taking the vitamins again because he had started to grow very restless and weary. These were the withdrawal symptoms caused by the addiction to the vitamins. I told the pastor to wait for a couple more days and stay strong through the withdrawals if he wanted his health back.

Two months later, the pastor came in looking bright and healthy. "You gave up the vitamin C and multi-vitamins, didn't you?" I asked. He smiled and said that it had been quite a journey. When I asked where his wife was, he told me she was too embarrassed to come because she did not believe me and got upset instead. He no longer had to take any more medications or insulin and was much healthier than before. He has since been taking vitamin E, which is good for *Soh Yang Ins*. He really had no idea that taking vitamins not fit for one's *Chejil* could do so much damage to one's body.

Harmful

A lady in her mid-fifties had been suffering from stomach and headaches for six months. Except for the congestion on her stomach walls, there was nothing odd about her health even after examining her stomach twice through endoscopy. Her digestion was fine and she was going to the bathroom regularly as well. The hospital just sent her off with some antacids but it did not help with her pain at all.

If there is nothing physically or internally wrong with the one's body but one still feels symptoms, it most likely has to do with what is being eaten. There is usually a habit of eating food that is bad for one's *Chejil*, or taking health products that are too strong.

She was a *Toh Yang Chejil* (*Soh Yang In*) and had a very fast pulse rate of 90 beats per minute. Her blood pressure was 130-180, which is in the normal range. During the consultation, I found out she had been taking vitamin B-Com for about a year which was the main cause of her ailment. Vitamin Bs in general are very bad for *Soh Yang Ins* because it strengthens an already strong digestive system, thus amplifying the imbalance between the organs. I explained this to her and told her to stop taking vitamin B-Com at once in order for the treatment to work. When she did not accept my explanation, I told her that she could go through my treatment once and then start taking the vitamins again to see what happens. I gave her the first acupuncture treatment and five days' worth of medication. The next day, she came back saying that her stomach felt a lot lighter and her head did not ache as frequently. Three treatments later, 90% of the pain had gone away, and after five more days of medication, she was cured. I advised her to only eat food and health products that were good for *Soh Yang Ins* and suggested vitamin E for strengthening the kidneys.

Like this case, I have had many *Soh Yang In* patients who suffer from stomach diseases due to the intake of vitamin B in its various forms. These products are only good for *Soh Eum Ins* who have very weak digestive systems.

IV

Chejil and Diets

"Results judge the value of theories"

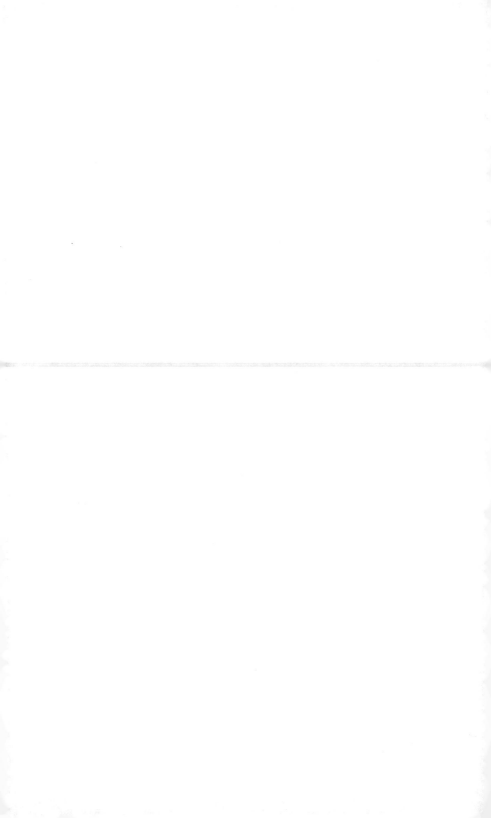

The *Chejil* Diet

People nowadays will try and do anything to lose weight. Regardless of one's age or sex, everybody is trying to figure out how to shed off a few pounds and it is not just an exaggeration when I say that they would do anything. Unfortunately, some people have actually died from being obsessed with weight loss.

There are countless methods of losing weight. One can either starve oneself, eat only meat (also know as the Emperor's Diet), just drink a lot of water, take diet pills, or even induce vomiting. These things can really endanger your health by causing side effects that can result in gaining weight rather than losing it.

If people select diet plans that fit their *Chejil*, however, it is possible to lose weight without damaging health.

The Emperor's Diet

The diet that primarily focuses on meat is good for everyone except *Tae Yang Ins*. The object is to stay away from carbohydrates and stick with meat and vegetables. However, the side effects of this diet can include excessive abdominal pain, headaches, diarrhea, and constant tiredness. This is, in large part, due to choosing foods not compatible with one's *Chejil*.

Different kinds of meats and vegetables are suitable according to each *Chejil*. For example, *Tae Eum Ins* can eat any kind of meat and root vegetables, but never fruit. *Soh Yang Ins* are better off with pork and maybe beef, but should never eat chicken or lamb. Unlike *Tae Eum Ins*, they should eat green leafy vegetables along with watermelon, melons, bananas, strawberries, and pineapple but never sour fruits such as apples, oranges, and mangos.

Soh Eum Ins should eat lamb and maybe beef but never pork. Vegetables are not good for them while sour fruits are ok. Diabetes patients should never eat fruit because it can raise the blood sugar level.

A woman in her early-forties came to me saying she wanted to lose weight. She was a *Soh Yang In*, so I told her she could try the Emperor's diet using pork or beef, egg whites only, and green leafs that are raw or steamed. I recommended this diet only for dinner, and after ten days, she called saying that she had lost six pounds, her constipation had gone away, and her back felt much better. I asked her how she did it, and she told me that for dinner, she would eat some of steamed beef, 1 egg white, and a small salad. If a *Soh Eum In* wanted to do this, he/she should eat either beef or chicken and not the egg white nor the salad. She gave me another call one month later saying she lost another seven pounds, which meant a total weight loss of thirteen pounds. Also, her back was completely healed and she was as healthy as she could be.

Vegetable Diet

Many people think that vegetables cannot be a cause for weight gain, but this is not true. There are people who eat a lot of vegetables but are still chubby and are not able to lose any weight. They often complain about headaches, dizziness, and most often about how they cannot lose weight even with vegetables. These are mostly *Tae Eum Ins* who still gain weight and get very sick from eating vegetables. Unless they stop eating them, nothing will be able to cure their sicknesses. *Tae Eum Ins* need to eat root vegetables such as carrots while *Soh Yang Ins* and *Tae Yang Ins* should eat green leaf vegetables.

Egg Diet

Lately, many people have started such a diet of eating only eggs for either all three meals or just for dinner. Some have given up due to heavy indigestion while others suffer from restlessness and dizziness despite the weight loss. If you are the right *Chejil*, this diet can work efficiently. This is only suitable for *Tae Eum Ins* and *Soh Yang Ins* if they eat only the egg whites. *Soh Eum Ins* and *Tae Yang Ins* are not fit for this method.

A man is his early-fifties who was getting treated for his sore knees asked me what he could do to lose some weight. He was a quite stout *Tae Eum In*, being around 5'5" tall and weighing 160 pounds. When asked how much he wanted to lose, he answered around ten pounds. I suggested a diet that would be safe for his health, easy to do, substituted only for dinner. He was interested and wanted me to tell him more about it. I told him to rotate each dinner between boiled eggs, well done meat, steamed carrots, and tofu. For his first dinner, he had two boiled eggs, a carrot, and a glass of water. Since he was still hungry, I told him to eat more eggs. He asked if it was okay to eat five eggs starting the second day. I told him that *Tae Eum Ins* could eat much more but since it could burden the stomach, it would be better to start off with two or three at first and lower the amount later on. A few days later, he told me he felt much lighter after having eaten two eggs and a carrot regularly. He lost ten pounds within three weeks, and since eggs can get very dull after a while, I told him it was alright to eat well cooked meat or tofu (warm or cold) instead. While one might think of replacing all three meals with the eggs or tofu in order to lose more weight faster, that kind of diet would need a serious consultation with the doctor in order to see if it would be harmful or not. To follow an economical, easy, and healthy diet, people should check their *Chejil* first to see what methods are good for them. In this case, only *Tae Eum Ins* should follow the egg diet.

Tofu Diet

As one of the very popular diet treatments, the tofu diet is only allowed for *Tae Eum Ins*. If *Soh Yang Ins* decided to follow this, they may damage their stomachs and experience other side effects such as hyperacidity, headaches, constipation, diarrhea, abdominal pain, and even skin infections. This diet is also not suitable for *Soh Em Ins* or *Tae Yang Ins*. *Tae Eum Ins* can get good results simply by eating tofu for dinner.

Fruit Diet

The fruit diet is as well known as the vegetable diet. Many people may suffer side effects, such as, stomachaches, hyperacidity, headaches, and abdominal pain. This is largely due to eating the wrong kinds of fruit that are not fit for one's *Chejil*. *Soh Yang Ins* should eat watermelon, melon, strawberries, bananas, and pineapple. Apples, oranges, tangerines, and mango are good for *Soh Eum Ins*. *Tae Yang Ins* are fine with almost every kind of fruit, while *Tae Eum Ins* should avoid this diet (Refer to "The Good and the Bad").

A woman in her late-30s came in interested in the *Chejil* diet. Although she did not look like she needed to lose weight, her goal was to lose ten pounds. She had tried many diets before but nothing changed but her health. She experienced more fatigue, headaches, constipation, and, insomnia. After hearing about the harmless and easy *Chejil* diet, she became very interested in learning more. I diagnosed her as a *Soo Yang Chejil* (*Soh Eum In*). She had a weak pulse rate of 70 beats per minute and she had regular constipation, so I recommended that she go on the fruit diet, specifically with apples and maybe oranges and mangos as well. Also, I warned her to never eat watermelon, strawberries, bananas, and pineapple since it could damage her body. I suggested that she eat the fruits for dinner with some water for a couple of days. After two weeks, she lost five pounds, was no longer constipated, and had better skin.

Soh Yang Ins interested in the fruit diet should eat the opposite of *Soh Eum Ins*, such as watermelon, strawberries, bananas, and pineapple. Regardless of the *Chejil*, diabetes patients should make sure to talk to a professional about eating any kind of fruit.

Potato Diet

The potato diet can be done by either substituting only one or all three meals with potatoes. Many people think potatoes are a bad diet product since they are high in carbohydrates, but many people, *Soh Eun Ins* and *Tae Eum Ins* in particular, have gotten good results from it. *Soh Yang Ins* and *Tae Yang Ins* should not try this diet.

Watermelon Diet

This is currently one of the most popular diets. It can help in massive weight loss, but *Soh Eum Ins* and *Tae Eum Ins* will suffer from indigestion, headaches, dizziness, gastric stomach. On the other hand, *Soh Yang Ins* can go along with this method without any negative side effects.

I hope for people to find their own *Chejil* diet that will really help them in numerous ways. Eating at least one dinner with the right kind of food will result in healthy and successful weigh loss.

The Celebrity *Chejil* Diet (1)

A while ago, there was an article about diets done by many celebrities such as Kim Sun Ah, Um Jung Hwa, Kim Hee Sun, and Hwang Shin Hae. It could have just been a mere coincidence but when I read the article, it was actually talking about the *Chejil* diets I have just explained. I am not quite sure how each of these celebrities did it, but it seemed like they all found the right diet for their *Chejils* and really gained success from it.

From the methods I have explained, singer Um Jung Hwa and actress Kim Sun Ah ate only half of their usual amounts and drank water whenever they were hungry. They carried around a bottle of water everywhere they went and drank it constantly. Drinking twice the regular amount of water, which has no calories, will clean out the organ's waste, making the skin more clear. The two made sure to drink as much water as they could, except half an hour before and an hour after each meal.

From my guess, and according to their physiques and personalities, they were both *Soh Yang Ins*. The water diet is healthy for *Soh Yang Ins*, who are recommended to drink cold water even on empty stomachs. If *Soh Eum Ins* try this method, they will suffer various side effects. This is because they have naturally low body temperatures and weak bodies, and do not like to drink a lot of water. If they were forced to drink too much water, it could cause harmful side effects.

The Celebrity *Chejil* Diet (2)

I want to talk about the honey diet that was made popular by actresses Kim Hee Sun and Hwang Shin Hae. Whenever their bodies felt heavy, they would mix some natural honey into warm water and drink it whenever they could. After drinking the honey tea for all three meals for three straight days, they would then eat a small amount of soup or a piece of bread, and would then recover and finish the diet off with either vegetables or tofu. The honey was to be 100% natural and the diet was to be done only once a month, never going over three days in duration.

In my opinion, it seemed like they were both *Soh Eum Ins*, thus the reason the honey worked. Honey along with warm water is good for *Soh Eum Ins*, so this can be a good diet plan for them. They need to make sure to eat the right kind of soup and bread to recover on the last day. If you are a *Soh Yang In*, the honey diet will only give you side effects such as indigestion, sour stomach, constipation, fever, tinnitus, rashes, arthralgia, and headaches. Other *Chejils* can also suffer from the same things but not as severly.

The Celebrity *Chejil* Diet (3)

"Ice Cream Can Make You Lose Weight," was the title of an article in a magazine called *Prevention*. This was a new diet plan that instructed people to eat low- fat ice cream as a meal. The other two meals were to consist of normal portions without any overeating. This diet plan, however, was not for everyone. There are people who do not like ice cream or if they do eat it, they get upset stomachs, head-aches, and even diarrhea. This happens mostly to *Soh Eum Ins* and *Tae Yang Ins*. So this diet should only be used by *Soh Yang Ins* and maybe even *Tae Eum Ins*.

This also goes for the yogurt diet done by actress Park So Hyun. Like ice cream, yogurt is a dairy product that is suitable for *Soh Yang Ins* and *Tae Eum Ins*. Just because a famous celebrity has succeeded using a certain diet plan does not mean it will be the same for everyone else. People need to choose the ones that are best for their *Chejil*.

This is an excerpt about the state of health taken from teacher Huh Joon's famous *Dong Eui Bo Kam*:

Hyung Jang Bool Kuep—people with smaller phy-siques are healthier than people   with bigger phy-siques; *Bi Bool Kuep Soo*—thin people are healthier than overweight people; *Dae Bool Kuep So*—people who eat little will live longer than people who eat a lot.

The conclusion: It is never healthy to overeat and become overweight.

Many medical professionals say, that weight loss is required for a long and healthy life. Losing weight requires very strong willpower and determination. Recklessly trying to lose weight is a bad idea that can easily damage one's health. Many people lose their health instead of weight while trying out new diet methods that were successful for other people. Just because it worked for certain people does not mean it will work for everyone. Of course, only people who have succeeded in their own diets recommend it to others. So, then, why do you think the same diet plans can work for one person but not for the other people? This is because of the differences in *Chejil*. Thus, diet plans for your health and beauty need to be carefully considered, according to one's *Chejil*, before anything is done.

The Emperor's Diet
for Each *Chejil*

The protein diet, also known as the Emperor's diet, was first introduced to the world by Yi Gun Hee, owner of the Samsung Company. A few years ago, Mr. Yi announced his successful weight loss through this method, and from then on, it became one of the most popular diets. Just like how the Emperor eats, this diet involves eating meat as a primary source. Unlike other diet plans where one eats very little or nothing at all, the Emperor's diet can be achieved by eating as much as one wants while still managing to lose weight. While other diet plans tend to be a failure for most people since it requires so much determination and willpower, this diet has a high success rate. The drawback is that there are limits as to what one may eat.

The Emperor's diet requires a lot of protein, like meat, with little or no carbohydrates. Carbohydrates turn into glucose once inside the body, and when that happens, a part of it will get burned off as energy while the other part remains and becomes fat, thus the weight gain. If no carbohydrates are taken in, the fats within the body burn off as a last resort to make energy, thus a catalyst for weight loss. This is why many diet plans require eating little or no carbohydrates. The same goes for the Emperor's diet, and like any other diet, this also does not provide good results to everyone. While some can achieve their goals without any harm, many experience side effects instead. For example, people may get indigestion, bloating, tiredness, constipation, dizziness, higher cholesterol level, osteoporosis, arteriosclerosis, and halitosis. These are usually caused by wrong food choices during the process. *Tae Eum Ins* and *Soh Yang Ins* can lose weight without any worries because meat is suitable for their *Chejils*. *Soh Yang Ins* just need to be careful to avoid chicken and lamb, while *Tae Eum Ins* are fine with almost all kinds of meat. Most people like to eat vegetables along with meat, so it is also important to choose the right kinds of vegetables. *Tae Eum Ins*, for example, need to eat root vegetables while *Soh Yang Ins* are better off with green leaf vegetables. This precaution goes for other food items as well, and is also what makes a healthy and successful diet for each of the *Chejils*. The bad thing about the Emperor's diet is the potentially excessive weight gain after the diet is over. This occurs because during the diet, one reduces the intake of fat while increasing the size of the stomach from the increased consumption of meat. The most efficient way to lose weight without any negative side effects is to eat food that best suits one's *Chejil*. This is the basis of the *Chejil* diet. I truly hope that you will find the right diet plan for yourself that will give you great and healthy results.

V

CHEJIL
AND
SICKNESS

*"If you know your Chejil, both general and incurable
diseases can be healing."*

Irritable Bowel Syndrome (1)

Seoul was quite chilly when I went to visit in late November of 1999. When I arrived at my in-laws' place that afternoon, my father-in-law was suffering from a very painful stomachache. My mother-in-law told me he had been having the stomachaches ever since Thanksgiving (*Chu Sok*), and that they had become worse at nights. He also could not go to the bathroom, often felt dizzy, and had a hard time breathing because his chest felt too stuffy. After a visit to the hospital, he found that he had irritable bowel syndrome.

He had a weak but fast pulse of 85 beats per minute. I diagnosed him as a *Tae Eum In* (*Mok Eum Chejil*) and gave him the appropriate acupuncture treatment. He felt his stomach become lighter and his head clearer. The hospital told him to eat meals packed with fiber, such as Chinese cabbage, spinach, fish, and fruits, and absolutely no meat. It was just as I thought, so I asked him if that diet had done him any good. He told me that it felt like it was working at first, but as time went by, his health started to deteriorate more and more. I explained to him that *Tae Eum Ins* like him who had short and weak large intestines needed to stay away from leafy green vegetables and fruit, which will actually worsen irritable bowel syndrome. From that day, I told him, he needed to start eating primarily meat.

During a conversation between family members, I could not help but to talk about my father-in-law's intestine check-ups. The check-up, which usually lasts fifty minutes, lasted only ten minutes for him because of the short length of his intestines. The next morning, my father-in-law was happy that he was able to sleep quite comfortably without dizziness or stomach pain. From then on, the whole family started eating mostly meat. A few days later, I accompanied both of my in-laws to Los Angeles, where I gave my father-in-law the appropriate acupuncture treatments as well as medication. He was completely cured by his tenth day in LA, and improved so much that he and his wife started taking long walks. Had my father-in-law kept eating vegetables, fish, and fruits, his sickness would have gotten worse and the healing process would have taken much longer.

The above story is very different from the conventional wisdom of today's medical theories. Thinking that vegetables and fruit are always required to treat stomachaches is quite a misconception. From the *Chejil* medicine point of view, there are as many people who need to eat meat as much as fruits and vegetables to heal their sicknesses. If you or anyone you know suffers from extreme stomach pains, such as those that come with irritable bowel syndrome, and if no treatment seems to work, checking your diet is an appropriate step to take. If you have been eating mainly vegetables and fish but the pain is still lingering, it would be wise to try eating more meat and less of everything else. This works the other way around as well. In this way, many sicknesses that cannot be cured through modern medicine can be treated through *Chejil* medicine. It is my hope that people will start understanding and embracing this more.

Irritable Bowel Syndrome (2)

A missionary from my wife's church came back to LA after working in Mongolia, and about two months after his return, he started having serious stomach problems along with constipation. He could not sleep at night, making it hard for him to live his daily life. The medication prescribed from the hospital was not helpful at all, and the pain seemed to get worse. My wife suggested that he come into my office for treatment, and since there were no improvements on his sickness, he finally decided to come for a visit.

He seemed like a traditional *Tae Eum In* with a short and chubby stature. My prediction was correct, and after the first acupuncture treatment, his stomach felt much lighter. I prescribed him some medicinal decoction and gave him a list of food he should and should not eat. When he started reading down the list, he looked at me suspiciously, saying that the food he should not be eating was what the hospital specifically wanted him to eat. They instructed him to eat high-fiber foods, such as vegetables and fish but never meat. From modern medicine's point of view, it is obvious to eat products high in fiber in order to treat stomach pain. However, *Tae Eum Ins* (*Mok Eum Chejil*), like this missionary, should avoid fiber and start eating more meat even though they have trouble with bowel movements. In other words, vegetables (maybe with the exception of root vegetables) and fruit are very harmful for them.

The answer lies in what caused his irritable bowel syndrome. While living in Mongolia, he consumed a lot of meat. When he came back to LA, he decided to eat more vegetables and fruit in order lose some weight and to be healthy again. He ate salads and fruit for dinner everyday, but after a while, his body started to swell up instead of becoming more lean. He also began to get restless as he started experiencing stomach aches. After about two weeks, his stomach pains grew worse and worse to the point where he could not even go to the bathroom anymore. This is what happens when *Tae Eum Ins* start to eat too many green leafy vegetables and fruit. The *Mok Eum Chejils* especially need to be careful about this because of their short and weak big intestines.

The next day, my patient came back, saying that it had been a long time since he had slept as comfortably as he had the night before. I gave him another acupuncture treatment along with oriental medication and told him to come back the next day. On the fourth day of his visit, the stomach pains had practically disappeared and his bowel movement improved. He received his last treatment, and I sent him off with ten more days' worth of medication. His stomach completely recovered just by eating meat—the opposite of conventional medical wisdom.

The insistence on eating only fruits and vegetables for stomach pains—is this really necessary? How many people would actually believe that stomachaches could be treated by eating meat but no vegetables at all? If you experience any discomfort from eating too much greens and fruit, it is highly probable that you are a *Tae Eum In*. *Tae Eum Ins* suffer from various side effects such as tiredness, serious stomach pains, constipation, migraines, skin infections, and different allergies if they start eating vegetables and fruit in hopes of enhancing their health. That is why irritable bowel syndrome is becoming so hard to treat with modern medicine and why so many people suffer from it. The main problem is that people do not have the slightest clue that the food they are consuming is the main reason for all their pain and sickness.

If you are experiencing discomfort in the body despite constantly eating vegetables or fruit, stop eating them immediately and see if the discomfort subsides. *Tae Eum In* females, especially, should be careful because their skin may react strongly and they may become discolored in the face when eating too many greens and fruits. More than 80% of my patients who have experienced irritable bowel syndrome have been *Tae Eum Ins*, so this tells you how important it is to eat the right kinds of food that fit your *Chejil*.

A Few Reasons for Constant or Increasing Blood Sugar Level

A. Taking vitamins not suitable for one's *Chejil*

Vitamins B and C can hinder the regulation of blood sugar levels for over 90% of all diabetes patients. If the regulation seems to be inconsistent despite the regular intake of diabetes medication, one should take precaution and check the kinds of vitamins he/she is taking. For a few, even vitamin E can be harmful for their blood sugar levels. This is why multi-vitamins are never helpful for diabetics. Various minerals can also be a problem.

B. Taking nutrients not suitable for one's *Chejil*

This is the same situation as above. If you are taking nutrients not fit for your *Chejil*, your blood sugar level can easily increase regardless of taking the appropriate diabetes medication.

C. Taking dietary supplements not suitable for one's *Chejil*

There are many kinds of dietary supplements available today. If the one you decide to take does not suit your *Chejil*, it can be a major problem in regulating your blood sugar level. Some people can take the same supplements without any problems while others can experience a highly increased blood sugar level.

D. Applying folk remedies not suitable for one's *Chejil*

E. Eating grain rice not suitable for one's *Chejil*

Eating rice with mixed grains can also increase your blood sugar level. It is wise to choose the right grains for your *Chejil* when you want to regulate the blood sugar level. Brown rice can give good results for *Soh Eum Ins* but can have bad effects for *Soh Yang Ins*. However, barley is a good choice for them, while it is bad for *Soh Eum Ins*.

F. Eating fruit

Fruit is not good for almost all diabetes patients. Even tomatoes can raise the blood sugar level for some people. However, there are situations in which bananas and strawberries will not do any harm for *Soh Yang Ins*.

G. Excessive stress

H. Eating food items containing sugar

These are mostly seen in western foods but can also be found in foods we do not think contain sugar, such as bean paste soup (*Dwen jahng jjigae*) served in Korean restaurants. They do this to give more flavor to the dish. If you eat foods like this without knowing the actual contents of it, the blood sugar level will inevitably rise.

I. Drinking tea not suitable for one's *Chejil*

Many teas that are known to be healthy can be the cause of elevated blood sugar level. This may seem rather strange, but if it does not suit you, it will result in bad side effects.

- When blood sugar level regulation does not go too well or it suddenly increases, it usually has to do with one of the above situations. To specifically figure out the problem, try quitting the food or products you may be taking for a couple of days and compare the blood sugar levels between the two time frames.
- Normal blood sugar levels:
  On an empty stomach: Below 120
  2 hours after meals: Below 160

Common Theories of Diabetes that are Untrue

Brown rice is the most popular item recommended for diabetics nowadays. Maybe that is why it is so well known to people and is increasingly available in restaurants. Also, various dietary supplements and other food items contain brown rice as the main component.

Recently, however, professionals are creating confusion among many diabetes patients telling them to stay away from brown rice or anything that contains it. It was a recommended food item that people ate when they got diagnosed with diabetes, but now people are saying that brown rice should not be consumed since it can have harmful effects. When people come in to my office to ask me about this, I answer that both theories are correct. This is because some have suffered from increased blood sugar levels while others have gained good results from eating brown rice.

Brown rice has warm qualities and will strengthen the stomach as well as the spleen. This is why *Soh Yang Ins* who already have strong digestive systems should stay away from it since it can raise blood sugar levels. On the other hand, brown rice helps out *Soh Eum Ins* who have cold and weak digestive systems. This is why I tell people that both theories concerning brown rice are correct.

Another example is when people recommend tomatoes

to treat diabetes. As with brown rice, there have been many concerns about eating tomatoes nowadays, which has created confusion among many people. This is because some people may experience negative results while others benefit from it. In *Chejil* medicine, tomatoes are good for *Soh Eum Ins* but not for *Soh Yang Ins*. People who tend to throw up bile when they eat tomatoes or drink tomato juice are most likely *Soh Yang Ins* or *Tae Eum Ins*. Many think that tomatoes will not affect the blood sugar level because it contains only a small amount of sugar, but this is a misconception.

If the blood sugar level of someone with diabetes does not seem to decrease after eating brown rice or dietary supplements made from it, he/she should stop eating them for a while and check the blood sugar level again. If the blood sugar goes down at that point, that means brown rice is not fit for that person. Eating it again would not be a good choice. On the other hand, if the blood sugar level remains the same as before (still high), that means something else is at work.

Beans are the same way. No matter how much you hear that rice with beans or tofu is good for you, this combination is very harmful for *Soh Yang Ins*, who get stomach aches with acidic belching, diarrhea, and excessive gas when they do eat it. Soy bean milk and other dietary products made of beans are also very bad for them. *Tae Eum Ins* experience the opposite affects, however. Eating beans will comfort their stomachs and they will experience regular bowel movements. If you become healthier and experience decreased blood sugar level by eating beans or bean products, you are most likely a *Tae Eum In.* Products that are known to be good for diabetes need to be chosen according to one's *Chejil* in order to achieve better health and lower blood sugar levels.

A *Tae Eum In*'s Cholesterol

A Middle Eastern man in his forties came into my office saying that he was experiencing anxiety problems and insomnia. He told me that his cholesterol level was over 400 when he tested his blood two years ago. His doctor told him to stop eating meat and start consuming more vegetables, fish, and fruits in order to decrease his cholesterol level. A couple days later, he started to get anxious and could not sleep at night. The symptoms became worse as his muscles and legs started to weaken and he began to feel pain in his elbows, wrists, fingers, and knees. Although his cholesterol level had gone down to about 220, the anxiousness grew worse, his palms and feet started to heat up, and his stomach became very queasy. The results were still normal, however, after an electrocardiogram and other various tests.

I began to examine him and diagnosed him as a *Mok Yang Chejil* (*Tae Eum In*). Keeping in mind that his doctor had recommended a diet of vegetables and fish, I instructed him to eat the opposite of that, especially being sure not to eat any green leafy vegetables. At this, he was very surprised and did not understand why I would say such a thing. So, I explained *Chejil* medicine to him—how people experience different effects from eating the same kinds of food because of different *Chejils*. The more I explained, the more he seemed to understand what I was talking about. He told

127

me he would do as I say. People who are *Mok Eum Chejils* (*Tae Eum In*) have strong livers but weak lungs, so they need to eat more meat and root vegetables and never green leaf vegetables. I gave him the list of food he should or should not eat and he agreed to stop taking the cholesterol medication for a while. A week later, he experienced positive results and after two weeks, he told me he felt much better. The anxiousness, in particular, went away very rapidly, and he was also able to sleep well at night. A month later, all his symptoms disappeared and his cholesterol level went down to 182—he was completely cured. The patient was worried that the symptoms would reappear, so he told me that he would come in at least once a week as a preventative measure. Even now, after a couple of months, he still comes in once a week to get his regular check-ups. He has maintained his diet of eating meat and never green leafy vegetables. As a result, his cholesterol went down again to 180. He continues to be amazed at how strange it is to have his cholesterol level lowered just by eating meat—something he would have never thought of. He is now a strong believer of *Chejil* medicine and always makes sure to check with me to see if new health products or foods he wants to take will be suitable for him or not.

Articular-Rheumatism Treatment

A lady in her early sixties came in last June and the moment she came in, I could see that something was wrong. She had a very unnatural walk and seemed very annoyed for no particular reason. It turned out that she had been suffering from articular-rheumatism for twenty-five years.

Her whole body ached, especially the joints in her hands, and she also had severe migraines. The pain in the joints of her shoulders, elbows, wrists, fingers, knees, ankles, and toes was so excessive that she would cry. The pain would keep her up at night and prevented her from taking care of her young grandson during the day. Although she had been consistently taking the appropriate medication and pain killers, her back still ached too much and she just could not stand it anymore.

I diagnosed her as a *Soh Yang In* and gave her the appropriate acupuncture treatment as well as a list of foods she should and should not eat and told her to come back the next day. When she came back, she told me that she was able to sleep much better than before, so I gave her another acupuncture treatment and also prescribed her some *Dok Hwal Ji Hwag Tang* (獨活地黃湯). After two weeks of treatment, her pain went away enough for her to sleep much more comfortably even without taking the medications given by the other doctor. She told me she had not slept so well in over twenty-five years, and after another week, the pain disappeared altogether, including the migraines. After six months, her fingers straightened out, enabling her to cook and do other things she could not before. She could even run without feeling any pain in her legs, and the best news of all is that there were no signs of rheumatism in her system when she got her blood checked again.

Articular-rheumatism is known to be a very serious and devastating disease that is frequently incurable. The main characteristic of this sickness is that the pain spreads symmetrically, and as time goes by, the cartilage gets damaged, causing a deformation in the joints in small areas like the fingers. It can become deformed in very noticeable ways and can affect the movements of the hands and other places as well. The actual and specific cause of this disease is not known yet, but we do know that it is a sickness that affects the whole body as an autoimmunity disease.

The immune system in our body protects from external viruses and bacteria. However, the system can become defective and work in reverse, against our own bodies, causing various diseases known as autoimmune diseases.

Autoimmune diseases can be classified into two categories—ones that attack one specific organ, or ones that attack the whole body, such as articular-rheumatism. Just as the cause of lymphatic disease lies somewhere outside of the lymph nodes, the origin of articular-rheumatism may come from a place other than the joints. Rheumatism can affect other parts of the body like the lungs, blood vessels, nervous system, and eyes. Arthritis is only a partial expression of diseases that affects the whole body. There is no perfect treatment for articular-rheumatism and medication usually consists of painkillers and anti-inflammatory pills. Since these are very strong in nature, they can cause major side effects to the digestive system, liver, and kidneys. Carcinostatic substances and steroids are also used in the worst cases.

In oriental medicine, articular-rheumatism is also known as *Bi Jeung*, supposedly caused by the attack of wind, cold, and moisture in the joints and meridian pathways, which then affects blood circulation. Thus, the three attackers are treated through acupuncture and medication to get blood circulation back to normal, thus strengthening the immune system.

The treatments of eight *Chejil* Medicine is amazing in that it strengthens the immune system by regulating the imbalance between the organs, potentially curing illnesses thought to be incurable. Every time I think or hear about cases like this, I always remember to thank and honor the creator of *Chejil* medicine, Yi Jae Ma and the creator of the acupuncture treatments and 8 *Chejil* Medicine, Kwon Do Won.

Treatment of Vocal Cord Tumors

I have a friend who used to be a photographer for the *Korea Times* in Los Angeles, along with assuming the directorships of other papers. Because of all his press duties, he had opportunities to meet and know many people. With very kind features and a husky voice, he was quite stout and of normal height. He appeared a bit old for his age and was a very faithful father and husband. Since he worked near my office, he would stop by once in a while to talk and catch up on old times.

One day this friend of mine came into my office worried about a small tumor in his vocal cords, asking me if oriental medicine could be of any help. His voice was almost like a whisper. His throat had begun to hurt three to four years ago, and had gotten to a point where he could not even talk because he was in so much pain. Since it had become so frustrating for both him and others around him, he finally went to an ear, nose, and throat doctor and unfortunately found out he had two small lumps on both sides of his vocal cords. The doctor told him he needed a biopsy and then a surgery, but he preferred oriental treatments instead.

His treatments began on January 8, 2002. The first day, I examined his *Chejil* and gave him an acupuncture treatment as well as a list of recommended foods. Starting the second day, I prescribed him medication and continued with the acupuncture treatments. After the third treatment, he told me that his throat felt much better and his voice became stronger than before. He came back consistently for treatments and as time went by, the condition of his throat improved even more. During the second week of treatments, he said his throat started to tickle and a few days later, he gave me a call with an urgent voice saying that something strange happened to him that day. It turned out that a small piece of flesh was coughed out while he was trying to cough out some phlegm. After a while, another piece got sneezed out of his nose when it started to get really itchy and stuffy. When I asked him how his throat felt, he answered in a loud voice that it felt very light and clear. I told him that that was a very good sign and recommended that he get some rest and come back the next day. After hanging up, I thought about Dr. Kwon, the creator of the 8 *Chejil* theory and could not help but to respect and honor him once again.

When my friend came in the next day, he was in a very good mood. When he went back to the doctor after one month of treatments, the two lumps were nowhere to be found. In other words, it had disappeared in only a month's time. He could not thank me enough and was so amazed at the results that *Chejil* medicine had brought him.

This *Chejil* theory has very drastic and fast effects that can cure many kinds of diseases, and once again, I cannot help but to thank and honor the work and legacy of Dr. Kwon.

Glaucoma

A very tall Caucasian couple in their early seventies came in to my office. They both had very kind and warm features and were very stylish. When I asked them why they came in, the husband told me about the pain in his elbows from playing golf, and the wife said she had been suffering from glaucoma for over twenty-five years.

Talking specifically about the wife's situation, the increased pressure in her eyes made it very difficult for her to see in general; colors were especially hard for her to see. She also had a narrow visual field. For example, her visual field was 50% less than normal. She could not tell green from gray, and her eyes became easily fatigued from reading. I started to examine her and found out that she was a *Mok Yang Chejil* (*Tae Eum In*), with a strong liver and weak lungs. I told her to immediately stop taking the multi-vitamin and vitamin C she had been taking and told her to replace them with vitamins A and D. When she asked me why, I explained the relationship between various vitamins and different *Chejils* to her. The couple seemed to understand what I was saying, and after I specifically explained some more, I gave her a list of foods she should or should not eat and warned her to never eat green leafy vegetables. I tried to explain why this was appropriate but she was not completely convinced and just wanted to go on with the treatments.

About three days later, the condition of her eyes and body improved greatly and she was more comfortable than before. However, after another two weeks, she said that she needed to talk to me about something. She told me that when she got her blood tested two weeks ago, her cholesterol level was 290 so the doctor told her to stick strictly to vegetables, fish, and fruits, and never meat. She did not know whose directions to follow—her doctor's or mine. It felt like she wanted to agree with her doctor rather than me, so I decided to stop the treatment for awhile and told her to follow the other doctor's orders and to come back if her cholesterol level was still high. Then I once again emphasized how harmful it is for *Mok Yang Chejils* to eat vegetables and made sure that she called me if her eyes or anything else got worse.

Ten days later, I got a call from the woman's husband saying that his wife wanted to start the treatments with me again. As it turned out, eating vegetables and forgoing meat only made her eyes and health much more worse than before. When she came back and resumed the treatments while eating more meat than vegetables, her eyes became clear again and the fatigue went away as well.

One day, she came to me excitedly talking about her trip to the stadium the night before. She was finally able to see the whole view of the stadium without any discomfort and the grass looked greener than ever. Experiences like these, where the eight *Chejil* medicine theory is able to treat disease like glaucoma, is when I cannot help but to again thank Yi Jae Ma and Kwon Do Won and the wonderful work they have done.

Why Diseases Get Worse Even With Treatment

Even with the same sickness and the same kind of treatment and medication, some people become better while others get worse. In the latter case, it is usually due to the intake of vitamins, minerals, or other dietary supplements that are not suitable for a *Chejil*. Common folk remedies can also be a problem. If one's health is not improving even with constant treatment, it is wise to pay a visit to the doctor to see which supplements are beneficial and which are not. To make it simple, try quitting all the extra supplements and see what happens. Folk remedies, such as eating grain rice, can also be an obstacle to one's treatment if it does not suit one's *Chejil*. *Soh Yang Ins* should never eat brown rice, glutinous rice, or rice with beans, while *Soh Eum Ins* should not be eating anything that contains barley. The same goes for various teas, raw food, and fruit juices. Even going to the sauna to sweat or drinking a lot of water can be harmful for some people. There are many times when a patient may feel pain and discomfort, only to find out that there is nothing wrong, according to the hospital. In such cases, doctors are not able to diagnose the specific causes and thus cannot prescribe the right kinds of medication. The doctor might just end up giving them pain killers, which can make the sickness even worse. Also, many patients in hospitals who have rare diseases with unknown origins are those who are taking too many supplements, thus negatively affecting their health. Supplements pertain not only to vitamins and minerals, but also to iron, magnesium, calcium, and others. This is why I think taking too many health products and other supplements without thinking about one's *Chejil* is the main cause of many rare diseases today.

A middle-aged lady came in with a skin infection in her chest area that caused itchiness and oozing sores. Even after a biopsy, the hospital was not able to diagnose the etiology of the infection. The medication prescribed by the hospital did not work. After I examined her, I discovered that the cause of the infection was due to health supplements she had been taking. Once she stopped taking them, the infection went away like magic. In cases like this, vitamins, minerals, and other products can be poison to our bodies if they do not fit our *Chejils*. It does not matter whether the ingredients are pure or not.

Most doctors think that stress is the main cause of sicknesses that are difficult to diagnose. The patients that I see, however, usually become sick because of eating the wrong kinds of products and foods, as opposed to stress. Be sure to check the kinds of supplements or folk remedies you are taking if you have a disease that can neither be diagnosed nor treated. Try to think of the time frames of when you first started eating various products and when you began to feel sick and try to figure out the relationship between those two time frames. No matter how good certain health products sound, it may be the cause of various diseases if taken by people whose *Chejils* do not fit with the ingredients. This is the basis and most important part of *Chejil* medicine.

VI

CHEJIL
AND
LIFESTYLE

"Healthiness can be achieved through knowing your Chejil."

The Spring Gala of Yi Hu Rak, The Old Country Man

The above title was published in a magazine very recently. Mr. Yi Hu Rak was the presidential secretary and head of the CIA during the third Republic under the reign of Park Jung Hee. He was known to be very influential and extremely well-informed in the behind-the-scenes story of all political wars. He was appointed the emissary for President Park Jung Hee before and after the "7.4 Declaration of North and South Association" in 1972. The conversation he had with Chairman Kim Il Sung at that time is still under a veil of secrecy, as is the behind-the-scenes story of his initializing the revitalizing reform during his time in the CIA in order to give President Park a chance for a prolonged one-man rule. After he was dismissed from his position in December, 1973, he fled the country with top secret files but decided to come back after negotiating with President Park. However, what was contained in those files is still a mystery even today. He was also important to various mystery cases, such as the murder of Mrs. Jung In Sook and the disappearance of the former head of the CIA, Kim Hyung Ook. In this way, Mr. Yi was one of the greatest powers during the third Republic and lived and witnessed history at that time. The honorary governor Kim Jong Pil even said a few years back, "The 1973 kidnapping of Kim

Dae Joong in Japan was committed by the head of CIA Yi Hu Rak. President Park and I had nothing to do with it." However, Mr. Yi has been avoiding the press for a while now, not talking about matters in public. He has refused all offers of writing an autobiography saying it is useless to talk about the past. Mr. Yi turned 79 this year and is starting to show symptoms of Alzheimer's disease, which is a big obstacle in trying to get more information on the history of the third Republic. Therefore, there is a high possibility that history will disappear without being told to anyone at all. He is currently living in a country house in Hanam, Kyunggido, without any connection to the outside world.

This is a short summary of the article about Mr. Yi:

"The doors of the country house owned by former head of CIA Yi Hu Rak in Hanam, Kyunggido, opened March 26 around 12:25 p.m. It's been awhile since he's come out to eat lunch at his favorite restaurant *Han Woo Ri*, only about 250 meters away. When the press started taking pictures upon his arrival at the restaurant, he showed severe discomfort telling them to stop taking his pictures at once. He was with four other people that day and decided to have bamboo tree rice Shabu-Shabu. According to the waitress, they ate the whole dish without any leftovers and even ordered more salad. Before his wife passed away, they used to come together frequently eating both lean meat (for his wife) and raw meat (for himself), but after his wife passed away about a year ago, he stopped ordering raw meat and started to eat more vegetables. On that particular day, he was in the restaurant for an hour, and when the reporter asked him about his recent health as he was coming out, he made an uncomfortable expression and called for his driver. While the driver went to retrieve the car, secretary Yi immediately paced toward the nearest hill off the road. The press interpreted this gesture as wanting them to leave him alone, but it turned out he had an emergency as his chauffer returned in a hurry to give him some toilet paper. After a while, secretary Yi came out with the assistance of his company and returned to his one and only safe zone— his house."

This was basically what the article was about and also what determined secretary Yi's *Chejil*. To simply state the conclusion, he is a *Tae Eum In*, and there are two reasons for this classification. The first is the fact that he had to go straight to the bathroom right after he ate, and the second is that he started to eat lots of vegetables after his wife's death. *Tae Eum Ins* are very sensitive and tend to get sour stomachs after eating vegetables, thus the sudden digestive reflex he experienced after unexpectedly running into the reporter. These are the usual and most commonly seen characteristics of *Tae Eum In* people.

It is Unhealthy
to Drink Too Much Water

"Drinking Eight Cups of Water a Day Isn't Always Good For You" was the title of a health column in a magazine. The Wall Street Journal article reported that the benefits of drinking a lot of water may be a misconception and that can be harmful to some people.

The commonly accepted guideline in terms of water consumption was the "8-8 rule," where drinking eight ounces of water eight times a day was the ideal water amount. Contrary to this rule, Heinz Bartin, a kidney specialist and professor at Dartmouth College, said that although many encourage drinking as much water as possible, there is no such scientific evidence for it. He had been researching the relationship between water and health for the past nine months. NAS also recently started a research group for their "8-8 rule" theory.

The conclusion is that our bodies might not need as much water as common theories recommend. The "8-8 rule" actually came out of research on soldiers in high altitudes and hospital patients. It is, therefore, not fit for normal everyday lives. If people drink too much water, they just feel the need to go to the bathroom more often. Moreover, for diabetes patients who take hormones preventing urination, the surplus of water will lower the sodium level in the blood stream, causing "water addiction" that can kill the patient. Many nutritionists have stated that drinking enough water to the point of not feeling parched is the right amount for people nowadays.

People are attempting to figure out whether drinking plenty of water as explained above is the right or wrong thing to do for one's health. Of course there may be some who benefit from drinking plenty of water, but most people do it because they think it is healthy or because everybody else is doing it. While some have achieved great results from it, others have experienced various side effects such as swelling, indigestion, and headaches.

There are those who drink only water through a "water diet" and experience excessive discomfort and weight gain, while others actually succeed with that diet without any negative side effects. The reason for all this is the difference in *Chejil*. When we look at the relationship between water and the various *Chejils*, *Soh Yang Ins* are usually the ones who become healthier by drinking plenty of water. There are people who drink water in the mornings on an empty stomach because they heard that it is good for them. It is mostly *Soh Yang Ins* with constipation, stomach diseases, skin diseases, and headaches who experience good results. However, there are also people who became more sick by drinking too much water. These are mostly *Soh Eum Ins* who do not like to drink water and become more sick from drinking too much of it. Some of them do not like to drink water even after meals and may dislike soups of any sort. They tend to drink only half a cup of water throughout the entire day. However, this does not affect their health adversely.

I sometimes worry and wonder about people who carry around water bottles and try to drink as much as they can. What if one is a *Soh Eum In* and he or she is actually drinking more and more water because of the side effects caused by drinking too much water? Whether drinking plenty of water is good for one's health or not is something that only *Chejil* medicine can answer for us.

Drinking Too Much Water May Cause Gastroptosis

Nobody was home when I came home early from work one Saturday evening. I was taking a nice nap when I got a call from the pastor's wife. I thought it was strange that she would call me at that time, so I asked her what was wrong. She asked me to come over quickly if I was not too busy. It turned out that a deaconess who had been suffering from a stomach disease for a long time needed my attention. Since she had never asked me for such a favor, I knew that this was an urgent situation. I told her that I would be there as soon as I could. I called my wife saying that we needed to go visit the pastor's place because of an emergency, and she said that she would come back home immediately. On our way there, my wife informed me that the deaconess had been giving out prayer requests about her sickness on the church bulletin for a while and was worried because it had become worse.

When we arrived there, the pastor, his wife, and the associate pastor were there with the deaconess and her mother. She was restlessly sitting on the sofa, and I heard that she had been suffering from indigestion, abdominal pains, stomach sores, hyperacidity, headaches, dizziness, and tiredness for the past three years. It had become so severe that she could not even get out of bed. Just a few weeks before, she had to go to the emergency room and stayed at the hospital for eleven days. They performed an endoscopy and discovered that she had inflammation in her stomach, which did not seem to be spreading. Other than that, everything else was perfectly normal. They assumed that it had to do with stress and sent her home. However, even after being discharged from the hospital, the sickness became so bad that the family started to worry about how long she had left to live.

The sickness started with indigestion about three years ago and continued to grow worse to a point where it affected her daily life. After that, she started having headaches with dizziness and soreness at the pit of her stomach. She also began to throw up acid, which made it hard for her to sleep. The pain grew so excessive that she started to stay constantly in bed.

After introducing myself quickly, I started examining her and asked if she had been taking any dietary supplements or doing any folk remedies at home. She told me that she regularly made potato and cabbage juice, rice soup, and just regular white rice, and that she also had been taking multi-vitamins, vitamin B, propolis, royal jelly, and aloe. Her overall body temperature was very low and weak. I diagnosed her as a *Soo Eum Chejil* (*Soh Eum In*).

I first gave her the appropriate acupuncture treatment and asked how she felt. The stuffiness in her chest had disappeared, and she was surprised by the quick results. I said that I would return the next day along with the necessary medication and asked her when she first began taking the aloe, multi-vitamins, and cabbage soup, since all three were harmful for *Soh Eum Ins*. She had started taking them much later than I expected, but I still warned her to stay away from them since it could worsen the pains and side effects.

Although I kept asking her many questions, I could not exactly figure out what was causing the sickness. I was not content with the fact that it was solely due to stress. As I was leaving, I asked her if she had been drinking large amounts of water. When she answered yes, I was very relieved to finally figure out that it had been the large amount of water that was causing all the problems. She informed me that she had been forcing herself to drink six or seven cups of water a day for the past four years because she heard that it was very good for her health.

The cause of all the pains and the "near-death" situation was water. I told her that *Soh Eum Ins* should not drink water much, and should stay away from soups and eat only dried food. She agreed and told me how hard it was for her to drink that much water every day. She also remembered that every time she drank it, her stomach did not feel very good.

The treatment for the deaconess ended in about three weeks, and she is now recovering. The gastroptosis she had was caused by drinking too much water for someone who already had a weak and cold digestive system. This was also the reason why so many other sicknesses such as indigestion and headaches occurred. What would have happened if she had kept on drinking so many glasses of water everyday? It gives me the chills just thinking about it. Like this, drinking too much water is not a healthy habit for everybody—*Soh Eum Ins* can become very sick.

Sweating and *Chejil*

There are two kinds of sweat in oriental medicine. One is called *Jah Han* and the other is called *Doh Han* . *Jah Han* refers to the regular sweat the body produces on its own during the day and can be sub-divided into *Ki Huh Jah Han*, *Hyul Huh Jah Han*, *Yang Huh Jah Han*, and *Sang Seup Jah Han* according to different origins. *Doh Han*, on the other hand, refers to sweat that is produced during the night only when the body is asleep. It is also known as *Chim Han* as well. *Doh Han* is caused by a lack of Yin and blood or by having too much dampness or heat in the liver . Sweating helps with excreting the waste from the body, but more importantly, it helps open up the sweat pores to let out the sweat, thus diffusing body heat. In other words, it controls body temperature. In oriental medicine, it also helps release energy from the body, which is why profuse sweating will make the body weak.

In recent years, many people have been trying various ways to sweat as much as possible for the sake of beauty and health. Whether working out at the gym, jogging, or going to the sauna, there are countless ways to "sweat it out." What relationship does sweat and *Chejil* have? There is a traditional Korean folk remedy of eating green bean sprout soup with lots of crushed peppers and then sweating underneath a very thick blanket in order to treat colds. Of course, this works for some, but it can also worsen the cold for others. There are people who become healthier by sweating at saunas or eating crushed peppers in soup. Then there are others who become sleepy, tired, and restless from the same activities. This is because some *Chejils* are meant to sweat excessively while others are not supposed to.

Tae Eum Ins and *Soh Yang Ins* are *Yi Yul Pyo Han Chejils*, which means that their bodies are warmer on the inside than on the outside, thus having more internal energy. On the other hand, *Tae Yang Ins* and *Soh Eum Ins* are *Yi Han Pyo Yul Chejils,* meaning they are cooler internally than externally, thus having more external energy. All this means is that *Tae Eum Ins* and *Soh Yang Ins* should sweat more often to balance the external and internal temperatures of the body. However, sweating will give the opposite effects for *Tae Yang Ins* and *Soh Eum Ins*—they will get tired, dizzy, weak, and sick. You might have heard of cases in which people pass out or get paralyzed from staying in saunas or hot tubs for too long. Of course blood pressure has much to do with it as well, but most cases are due to *Chejils* that are not meant to sweat.

Case 1

A woman who just gave birth four months ago came into my office wearing a very thick jacket in the middle of July. She had been suffering from severe chills even during the hot summer and had to use hot pad blankets, wear extra layers of clothing, and put on thick socks in order to sleep at night. Her hands and feet were always cold, and she had severe headaches, indigestion, and tiredness. as well. From the oriental medicine point of view, this patient had *San Hoo Poong* (being in the cold after birth) and had a very low body temperature. Women who get weaker bones from not taking better care of themselves after birth experience an accumulation of bad blood, or coldness (寒邪), and bad wind (風邪) during the *Ki Huh* (氣虛) and *Hyul Huh* (血虛) states, which is the main cause of *San Hoo Poong* coldness, thus giving pains and chills.

I diagnosed her as a *Soh Eum In* and asked how she took care of herself after giving birth. She told me that she had been sweating as much as possible after hearing that it would be good for her. That was the problem. Sweating will lower the temperature of the insides for *Soh Eum Ins* who already have very low inner body temperatures, which in turn will weaken their energy and thus cause indigestion, and headaches. along with tiredness and chills. Sweating is a good after-childbirth habit for *Soh Yang Ins* and *Tae Eum Ins*, but not for *Soh Eum Ins*. The patient was completely cured and healthy after ten days of treatment and stopped suffering chills. Like this, trying to sweat constantly for one's health can actually be the cause of many sicknesses if it does not fit one's *Chejil*. That is why it is also important to know which after-birth method is appropriate and healthy for you and your *Chejil*.

Case 2

A lady in her mid-fifties suffering from arthritis came into my office one day. She had been tired and restless for about a year and had been spending more time in bed and could not concentrate on anything else. She felt severe pain in her joints, and her fingers were very swollen. She could not bend her fingers or pick things up. I diagnosed her as a *Soh Eum In* and discovered that she had been taking hot baths regularly to sweat as much as she could. I told her to stop taking the baths immediately since it was the main cause of her arthritis. About three months later, the arthritis was completely gone and she no longer suffered from swollen joints.

Case 3

A foreign man in his early-forties came into my office through a Korean friend's recommendation. He had been suffering from tinnitus and told me that his ears had been ringing for two days and that it became so bad that he could not work or sleep. He was a *Soh Eum In* who became affected by going to the sauna too many times.

The patient owned a paint company and when one of his workers stopped coming to work, he had to do the work by himself for about a week. After work, he would go straight to the sauna to relieve the tiredness and stress he felt through that day and would sweat off as much as he could. After stopping his sauna visits, this patient also no longer experienced tinnitus.

There are many other cases where sweating has caused problems. Problems include indigestion, dizziness, headaches, bad eye sight, cold hands and feet, bad skin, chronic tiredness, and other unfortunate situations. You may have to re-think the sweating practice if you are doing it to treat any kind of sickness you may have, especially if you are a *Soh Eum In.*

Chejil Harmony Prediction

Before getting married, many Korean people go to a fortune teller to get predictions about their marital harmony and future with just giving their dates of birth (*Sah Ju* and *O-hang*) to the fortune teller. Of course it is quite hard to predict the actual future simply using birthdates, and many side effects can occur from it. That is why most people think it is better to do physiognomic readings rather that fortune telling. Physiognomic observing is probably very similar to looking at the mental image of a person since it reflects mostly what is on one's mind and thoughts. There are four popular sayings that relate to this—"*Jok Sang Bool Yuh Soo Sang*" (足相不女手相), "*Soo Sang Bool Yuh Gohl Sang*" (手相不如骨相), "*Kwan Sang Bool Yuh Shim Sang*" (觀相不如心相), and "*Gol Sang Bool Yuh Kwan Sang*" (骨相不女觀相). All these together mean "having good feet is no better than having good hands, having good hands is no better than having a good frame, having a good frame is no better than having a good facial appearance and having a good facial appearance is no better than having a good heart."

It may be confusing when I say that the harmony and health of one's family depends on the family's *Chejil*, but this is a very true statement. *Chejil* has a very close relationship to the happiness of a family. What two *Chejils*, then, would be most suitable for each other? The simple answer would be those that have the opposite weak and strong internal organs of each other. When two totally opposite *Chejils* meet, one's weak spot will be the other's strong point and vice versa, so the two can give each other the strong energy they have within them to make a healthier and stronger bond. There are many cases in which a couple becomes physically healthier after getting married. This is mostly because the two partners are total opposite *Chejils* of each other. *Chejil* harmony can be analogous to the principles of a magnet—only if the two opposite poles meet will there be an attraction between each other.

There are many married couples around us that never fight and are always picture-perfect happy. Such people are those who have met with the opposite *Chejils*. On the other hand, however, there are other couples who tend to fight constantly and even get divorced if it gets too bad. This is most likely because they are the similar or the same *Chejils*. From feeling unpleasant when lying under the same sheets to liking each other no matter where they are, from couples who can talk like best friends to those who try to pick a fight at every point, all are due to different *Chejil* harmonies within each couple. If the two are right for each other, they even like the smell of the other person without any disgust.

There was a health report that caught my attention recently from a Korean radio station. A geneticist did an experiment where he told four men to wear the same clothes without washing or putting on any deodorant for 48 hours and then asked each of them to take off their shirts and put them into four different boxes. Then, he gave the boxes to a group of women and told each of them to choose the best and worst smelling clothes. The results were that they chose the shirt worn by the man with the opposite genes from them as the best smelling shirt and vice versa. Putting the results of this experiment together, I can again say that two opposite *Chejils* will feel attraction for each other while two similar *Chejils* will not feel anything for one another at all. This is only a small part of *Chejil* medicine and also a grand start to diagnosing *Chejils* using the fundamentals of genetics, which is something I'm looking forward to.

The *Chejil* Revolution

If only knowing one's *Chejil* was as easy as knowing one's blood type, there would be major changes in every field known to man. People would not have to depend on hospitals as much because their sicknesses would be prevented by eating the right kinds of food and having a lifestyle fit for their own *Chejils*. Therefore, more and more *Chejil* medicine professionals will be needed while the need for other doctors will decrease. Also, a *Chejil* medicine department will have to be built in every medical school and may become a required course for all medical students. Many diseases that were incurable through modern medicine will be treatable through *Chejil* medicine, which will then elevate its status. For example, if a patient is sick but nothing can be found from the test results, it would be hard to find the appropriate medications or treatments to cure that disease. Or if something were to be found but treatment does not seem to work regardless of the right medications, the sickness can linger on or it may get worse. All these can be solved through *Chejil* medicine and thus, people will be able to live up to 120 years old without having to depend on any kind of medication.

Multi-vitamins will disappear as other vitamins get divided according to the different *Chejils*. Dietary supplements will also be divided in the same way so that *Soh Eum Ins* can have products made specifically for them, containing ingredients like ginseng and glutinous rice, while *Soh Yang Ins* can have barley.

Grocery markets will also divide their foods and other products according to *Chejil*, and restaurants will have titles such as *The Tae Yang In Restaurant* and the such. In restaurants where all *Chejils* are allowed to eat, they will prepare various kinds of rice and water fit for each kind of *Chejils*, such as brown rice, barley, green tea, and brown tea. This also goes for soft drinks since they would have different ingredients in each of them.

Clothing is also an issue—*Chejil* medicine will affect the textile industry to make different colored clothes for each *Chejil*: blues for *Tae Yang Ins*, whites for *Tae Eum Ins*, blacks for *Soh Yang Ins*, and yellows for *Soh Eum Ins*.

Architects would also build houses according to *Chejil*. For example, they would set up house signs that say things like "For Sale—4 beds (2 for *Tae Yang Ins* and 2 for *Tae Eum Ins*) & 3 baths." This is because each *Chejil* should sleep facing different direction according to where the sun shines and wind blows. The wall colors would also need to be different as well as the kind of blanket and pillow to use. Like this, *Chejil* medicine will affect almost everything in our everyday lives.

So when will all this actually happen? It is when just few drops of blood will be the only thing required to determine one's *Chejil*. I personally do not think that this will take a very long time. If and when that day comes, I believe that both teacher Yi Jae Ma and Kwon Dowon will be a major inspiration for everyone.

VII

TAE YANG IN
YI JAE MA

*"People will be able to live a long and healthy life,
treating their own sicknesses."*
Yi Jae Ma

A Greatly Expected TV Drama

The new drama "*Tae Yang In* Yi Jae Ma" is very popular among many Korean-Americans in Los Angeles. Many great articles and news about the show have been reported from the Korean media, which gave higher expectations and curiosity for many Koreans living in America.

While I was just as excited, I was also quite worried thinking that it was too early to introduce *Chejil* medicine since *Sahsang Medicine* is very different, if not contrary, from the conventional wisdom of modern medicine that everybody is so used to. If the show was properly produced, then it would surely prove the superiority of *Sahsang Medicine* along with the brilliant works of teacher Yi and also provide evidence for problems of other medical theories as well. Many medical cases that were not able to be solved through modern medicine would be fixed through *Chejil* medicine, giving it the superiority it deserves. Should this happen, the emphasis on the greatness of *Chejil* medicine would grow stronger as conventional medicine would weaken, then giving a negative effect to many of those working in that field. This in turn can prevent the drama from showing the true values of *Chejil* medicine in order to avoid complaints from the field of modern medicine, thus giving the wrong impression that *Chejil* medicine is not such a great deal after all. As someone who knows and respects *Chejil* medicine, I feel greatly worried that the show will turn out to be just talk and nothing more. As of now, I am half concerned and half excited to see the drama come to life as it can truly prove the greatness of *Sahsang Medicine* and everything that was done to create it.

I recommended this show to everyone saying that it would help them understand why mistakes are made in modern medicine as well as how to take good and appropriate care of themselves. I even said that it would be a huge loss if they decided not to see it and suggested to come see me if they could not understand something from the show.

Just as I predicted, many problematic subjects began to surface as soon as the drama started. There is a particular scene in which two men come to where teacher Yi Jae Ma worked, the *Soo San Won*, complaining about severe stomach pains one night. While Doctor Chun Sang Ok, who is somewhat like a boss to teacher Yi, examines the two men, teacher Yi starts asking them questions about what they ate for dinner that night. Both answer that they ate dried clam meat and tofu cakes. Dr. Chun concludes that they were suffering from bad stomach due to food poisoning and gives them *Dae Seung Ki Tang* (大承氣湯) as the appropriate medication. However, while one was totally cured through the treatment, the other unfortunately passed away the next day.

This is one case that many people probably did not understand. Why did one die while the other was cured after getting the same treatments for the same kind of sickness?

The answer was their difference in *Chejil*. Because of this, the medication had different effects—one's life was saved while the other was essentially poisoned. Therefore, different kinds of treatments are needed even for the same kinds of sickness according to their *Chejils*.

If you analyze the *Dae Seung Ki Tang* medicine shown from the above scene, it was supposed to cure constipation, indigestion, fevers, and anything else that pertains to increased heat. The main components, *Dae Hwang* (大黃) and *Mang Cho* (芒硝—sulphate of soda), are both cool in its chemical content, thus being harmful for *Soh Eum Ins* who already have a low body temperatures. There actually are some constipation medications being sold to the public, including *Dae Hwang*, that can make *Soh Eum Ins* have bad stomach aches and maybe even hemorrhoids if they decide to take them. It can be predicted that the person who died in the drama was most likely a *Soh Eum In* while the other person could have been either a *Tae Eum In* or *Soh Yang In*. No matter how healthy and great some food and products may look, it can lead to fatal consequences if taken by the wrong *Chejil*. This is the basic theory of *Chejil* medicine, and the very truth that can cure the incurable in modern medicine.

Since this drama can hugely affect all other medical theories in a very negative way, I am constantly worried about the possible negative outcomes. Nonetheless, I truly hope "*Tae Yang In* Yi Jae Ma" will become a big success without causing any troubles.

The TV Drama That Could Have Been Better

"*Tae Yang In* Yi Jae Ma" unfortunately ended with a quite disappointing finale, contrary to audience expectations. As I stated before, I was quite worried about the future of both modern and *Chejil* medicine as soon as I heard this show was to be aired on national television. This was because of the possibility of a big clash between the two medicines that are based on totally opposite bases and foundations.

Sadly, as predicted, problems came up after only a few episodes aired, and the broadcasting station received many complaints about it. Soon after the protests, the show began to focus more on teacher Yi's personal life rather than on *Chejil* medicine to avoid further conflicts. The show that kicked off with a grandiose start soon finished with an unexpected end, and the program itself became a waste. The sudden amends due to the heavy complaints were the main cause. As someone who has been keeping up with every episode with great anticipation, the show has become a huge disappointment. My worries had come true as people did not and could not understand the basis of *Chejil* medicine, and even if they did, they observed it as an alternative treatment method that derived from modern medicine.

I was hugely let down and disappointed. I am confident that *Chejil* medicine is a whole new kind of medicine whose founders should win a Nobel Prize. In the near future, *Chejil* medicine will be the center of focus for all other medicines to follow. But the question is, when? It will be the day when a baby's *Chejil* can be determined with 100% accuracy with just a few drops of his/her blood. When this day comes, I am certain that both teachers Yi Jae Ma and Kwon Do Won will be named as Nobel Prize winners. Teacher Yi says in his *Dong Eui Soo Sae Bo Won*, "100 years after my death, *Sahsang Medicine* will be known to all mankind and will be used worldwide as well."

Teacher Yi was born in 1837 and passed away in 1900 and just as he predicted, *Sahsang Medicine* is becoming very popular today as many books are being written for people to understand it better. More and more people are showing interest as they start reading the books and wonder what *Chejil* they are. Also, there is an increasing number of people who are starting to choose good and healthy diets and lifestyles according to their *Chejils*.

As someone who is in the field, I become very excited and ecstatic every time I see or hear people getting their "incurable" diseases treated through *Chejil* medicine. I also never forget to thank and honor the creator of *Chejil* medicine Yi Jae Ma and Kwon Do Won and their brilliant works. I strongly believe that a TV drama that tells the real and true values of *Sahsang Medicine* will soon air and become a big success not just for the producers, but for everyone in this world.

Made in the USA
San Bernardino, CA
31 March 2015